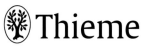

*For Anja and Heike—
without whose patience and support this book would
not have been possible.
Thank you!*

Trigger Points
and Muscle Chains
in Osteopathy

Philipp Richter, DO

Private Practitioner
Assistant Director of the Institute for Applied Osteopathy (IFAO)
Burg Reuland, Belgium

Eric Hebgen, DO, MRO

Private Practitioner
Königswinter, Germany

263 illustrations

Thieme
Stuttgart • New York

Library of Congress Cataloging-in-Publication Data is available from the publisher.

This book is an authorized and revised translation of the 2nd German edition published and copyrighted 2007 by Georg Thieme Verlag, Stuttgart, Germany. Title of the German edition: Triggerpunkte und Muskelfunktionsketten in der Osteopathie und Manuellen Therapie.

Translator: Sabine Wilms, PhD, Ranchos de Taos, New Mexico, USA

Illustrators: Malgorzata and Piotr Gusta, Champigny sur Marne, France; Christiane and Michael von Solodkoff, Neckargemünd, Germany

Richter, Philipp, 1960-
  [Triggerpunkte und Muskelfunktionsketten in der Osteopathie und Manuellen Therapie. English]
  Trigger points and muscle chains in osteopathy / Philipp Richter, Eric Hebgen ; [translator, Sabine Wilms].
    p. ; cm.
  Includes bibliographical references and index.
  ISBN 978-3-13-145051-7 (alk. paper)
1. Osteopathic medicine. 2. Manipulation (Therapeutics) 3. Muscles–Physiology. 4. Myofascial pain syndromes–Chiropractic treatment. I. Hebgen, Eric. II. Title.
  [DNLM: 1. Manipulation, Osteopathic–methods. 2. Myofascial Pain Syndromes–therapy. 3. Muscles–physiology. WE 550 R536t 2008a]
  RZ341.R5213 2008
  615.5'33–dc22
                  2008031519

Important note: Medicine is an ever-changing science undergoing continual development. Research and clinical experience are continually expanding our knowledge, in particular our knowledge of proper treatment and drug therapy. Insofar as this book mentions any dosage or application, readers may rest assured that the authors, editors, and publishers have made every effort to ensure that such references are in accordance with **the state of knowledge at the time of production of the book**.

Nevertheless, this does not involve, imply, or express any guarantee or responsibility on the part of the publishers in respect to any dosage instructions and forms of applications stated in the book. **Every user is requested to examine carefully** the manufacturers' leaflets accompanying each drug and to check, if necessary in consultation with a physician or specialist, whether the dosage schedules mentioned therein or the contraindications stated by the manufacturers differ from the statements made in the present book. Such examination is particularly important with drugs that are either rarely used or have been newly released on the market. Every dosage schedule or every form of application used is entirely at the user's own risk and responsibility. The authors and publishers request every user to report to the publishers any discrepancies or inaccuracies noticed. If errors in this work are found after publication, errata will be posted at www.thieme.com on the product description page.

© 2009 Georg Thieme Verlag,
Rüdigerstrasse 14, 70469 Stuttgart, Germany
http://www.thieme.de
Thieme New York, 333 Seventh Avenue,
New York, NY 10001, USA
http://www.thieme.com

Cover design: Thieme Publishing Group
Typesetting by Hagedorn Kommunikation, Viernheim, Germany

Printed in Germany by APPL aprinta druck, Wemding

ISBN 978-3-13-145051-7   1 2 3 4 5 6

Preface

The idea for this book originated many years ago. Practical experiences, reading specialized literature, attendance at seminars, and conversations with colleagues and specialists from other disciplines showed us time and again the significance of the locomotor system.

Daily clinical routine showed us in the course of years that the same lesion patterns tended to occur over and over. Years of intensive observation and investigation as well as thorough literature research confirmed that our observations agree with reality and are not just wishful thinking.

Not only osteopaths, but also posturologists and manual therapists, speak of motor patterns, using different explanatory models for the development of these patterns. In a course on muscle energy techniques, both *Dr. F. L. Mitchell Jr.* and *Dr. Ph. Greenman* referred to a universal pattern. Both agree on the existence of a universal pattern, because in the case of dysfunction in the motor system other body parts always adapt with identical patterns. Similarly, the entire organism follows certain patterns in physiology; examples include processes like walking or breathing. The common embryologic origin of all tissues, the connections of the connective tissue, and the organism as a hydropneumatic system all support this theory. The endocrine system is also a good example of holistic behavior.

The holistic principle, highly prized by the osteopath, as well as embryologic, physiologic, and neurologic axioms offers explanations for the origin of certain patterns. In our opinion, the nervous system and the myofascial structures play key roles in this process as organizer and as executing organ respectively.

We have compared different models of muscle chains and different osteopathic working models, looking for commonalities. Consequently, we have realized that all these models share a basic premise, but from different perspectives.

In this book, we present a model of muscle chains that is based on the two motor patterns of cranial osteopathy, namely flexion and extension. Because the organism consists of two halves, it has two corresponding chains of flexion and extension.

Littlejohn's model of the "mechanics of the vertebral column" and the "Zink patterns" of the American osteopath *Gordon Zink, DO* have inspired us to divide the torso skeleton into units of movement. Much to our surprise, we realized that this division into units of movement correlated closely with the division of neurologic supply of certain organs and muscles.

We provided both chains with muscles, understanding that this can only be incomplete and theoretical. We ask the reader to keep this in mind. Nevertheless, because the organism only recognizes motor patterns, but not individual muscles, this is somewhat irrelevant.

In the second part of the book, we present a number of treatment methods for the myofascial structures. For this purpose, we describe trigger point therapy in great detail because it is invaluable in clinic. We have purposely limited this presentation to the mechanical aspect of osteopathy because it is significant for posture and can therefore be applied in diagnosis.

For physiologic cranial dysfunctions, we have chosen a mechanical model to attempt an explanation. We have, however, refrained from presenting visceral dysfunctions in detail, in spite of the fact that they quite clearly follow the same patterns. Structural disturbances manifest in malposture through direct fascial trains and particularly through viscerosomatic reflexes. Following the holistic principle, the organs adapt to the "container," the motor system, in the same way that postural disturbances affect the location and function of the organs (adaptation of function to structure).

Our model of muscle chains is only a working model, just like many others; we do not lay claim to completeness. We were able to realize in clinic, however, that diagnosis as well as treatment of patients can become much more rational and effective when they originate in this perspective. This applies in particular to chronic and therapy-resistant cases.

Philipp Richter
Eric Hebgen

List of Abbreviations

ABD	Abduction	**OAA complex**	Occipitoatlantoaxial complex
AL chain	Anterolateral chain	**OM suture**	Occipitomastoid suture
ASIS	Anterior superior iliac spine	**OA joint**	Occiput-atlas joint
AIIS	Anterior inferior iliac spine	**ORL**	Otorhinolaryngology
ATP	Adenosine triphosphate	**PA–AP chain**	Posteroanterior-anteroposterior chain
CCP	Common compensatory pattern		
CNS	Central nervous system	**PL chain**	Posterolateral chain
CSC	Cervical spinal column	**PNF**	Proprioceptive neuromuscular facilitation
CSF	Cerebrospinal fluid		
CTJ	Cervicothoracic junction	**PRI**	Postisometric relaxation
CVB	Cervical vertebral body	**PRM**	Primary respiratory mechanism
EMG	Electromyography	**PSIS**	Posterior superior iliac spine
ERS	Extension-rotation-sidebending	**SAT**	Specific adjusting technique
FRS	Flexion-rotation-sidebending	**SBL**	Superficial back line
ILA	Inferolateral angle	**SBS**	Sphenobasilar synchondrosis
ISJ	Iliosacral joint	**SCM**	Sternocleidomastoideus/ sternocleidomastoid muscle
LSC	Lumbar spinal column		
LSJ	Lumbosacral junction	**SFL**	Superficial front line
LTA	Lower thoracic aperture	**TFL**	Tensor fasciae latae
MET	Muscle energy technique	**TLJ**	Thoracolumbar junction
MTP joint	Metatarsophalangeal joint	**TSC**	Thoracic spinal column
NCP	Non-compensated pattern	**TVB**	Thoracic vertebral body
NMT	Neuromuscular technique	**UCCP**	Uncommon compensatory pattern
NSR	Neutral position-sidebend-rotation	**UTA**	Upper thoracic aperture

Picture Credits

Contents

A

Muscle Chains
Philipp Richter

1 Introduction

1.1 The Significance of Muscle Chains in the Organism

The locomotor system, and in particular, the **muscle chains**, constitute the core of this book. The myofascial structures contribute to all bodily functions: emotional states manifest in muscular tension, muscular activity is necessary for all physical work, and even circulation, respiration, and digestion depend on an intact locomotor system.

Manual therapists, whether physical therapist, chiropractor, osteopath, or Rolfer, examine and treat the locomotor system differently and for different reasons. While physical therapists and Rolfers treat the musculoskeletal system primarily to remedy complaints (pain, malposture, and so on) in this area of the body, the chiropractor, and especially the osteopath, consider the myofascial system as a part of the organism that can be the cause as well as the result of dysfunctions or pathologies in other systems of the organism. Yet another professional group, the podologists or posturologists, as they are called in francophone countries, is aware of the negative impacts on the entire organism that can be caused by even minor shifting of weight or malpositions of the feet.

All bodily functions depend on well-functioning myofascial structures. The nervous system plays a coordinating and controlling role. To avoid overburdening the cortex, many activities are regulated by subcortical reflexes and behavioral patterns. Science has proven the existence of so-called viscerosomatic and somatovisceral reflexes, and emphasizes the significance of muscular imbalances, in particular of the paravertebral musculature.[79, 112]

The human organism functions in accordance with motion and postural patterns that involve the entire organism, just as all bodily activities always result from an interaction of all bodily systems. Osteopaths and chiropractors in particular, take advantage of this fact in diagnosis as well as therapy.

The segmental innervation of all body structures, as well as adaptive mechanisms in accordance with patterns, indicate affected structures. Often, sports injuries or pain in the locomotor system are the result of malfunctions in parts of the myofascial chains. Knowing the myofascial relations allows for diagnosis and makes a corresponding treatment possible. The osteopathic way of thinking offers an interesting explanation for the mechanisms that intervene in the formation of illness and its treatment.

1.2 The Osteopathy of Dr. Still

When Dr. Andrew Taylor Still presented his philosophy of therapeutics during a phase of rejecting the medicine practiced at that time, he called it **osteopathy**, knowing full well that this term had a different meaning among experts. In his desire to redirect medicine back to its origins, that is, to put the person at the center and natural laws in the foreground, osteopathy was the most accurate term to express the concept that illness (pathos) results from dysfunctions of the organism. Still accorded the locomotor system, and the vertebral column in particular, a central role. He had realized that all illnesses and functional disturbances were accompanied by restricted movement of the vertebral column. Osteopathy means the "pathos" that comes from the "osteo."[140]

Experience had taught Still that symptomatic treatment does not bring about cure. Only expert treatment of the cause was able to yield success. Still was convinced that illness begins with a disturbance of circulation and that the cause of this could be found in the connective tissue.[140] Consequently, this was where diagnosis and treatment had to take place.

The myofascial tissue is of particular significance because of its connective function (connective tissue) and its capacity to serve as a pathway for veins, lymph vessels, arteries, and nerves, as supportive tissue for organs and bones, and as a protective structure.[82, 140]

The nervous system and its surrounding liquid, the cerebrospinal fluid, are of perhaps even greater importance for Still than the connective tissue. The nervous system as control center and regulatory organ is in charge of all adaptive mechanisms between the individual body systems.

Still describes the **cerebrospinal fluid (CSF)** as perhaps the most important known element ("the highest known element") of the whole organism. In its constituents, it resembles the blood and lymph serum. It is connected to both of these fluids: with the blood via the plexus chorioidei and with the lymph via the peripheral nerves in the interstitial space. In addition to its supportive and nutritive functions for the central nervous system, Still, and especially his student Sutherland, accorded the CSF another special significance: together with the fluid, the "breath of life" infiltrates all body cells.[54, 140, 142, 143]

Personal events and experiences that Still had in his youth most likely played an important role in the creation of osteopathy. As physician, religious person, and son of a Methodist minister, Still had a close relationship with religion and God. This is reflected in his writings. To Still, God has given humans their health; illness is abnormal. For Still, it is the job of the osteopath to find health in the organism of the patient.

In his search for true medicine, Still was inspired by two opposite approaches: by spiritual healers and by bone setters. The spiritual healer represents the religious therapists who listen into the tissue and focus energy into the pathologic region through their hands. The "breath of life" will then take over the healing. On the other side are the bone setters who achieved equally great successes through physical manipulation.

In his osteopathic treatments, Still succeeded in uniting both of these approaches. His exact knowledge of anatomy, as well as his outstanding sense of touch, combined with his belief in the body's self-healing power and the *intention to help* made him an outstanding therapist. His anatomical and physiologic knowledge facilitated a precise visualization of structures. His sense of touch allowed him to detect tonicity in the tissue and hence apply the appropriate techniques in any given case. In Still the osteopath, the healer was united with the bone setter. He compared the human organism to a machine and the osteopath to a mechanic who repaired the mechanics of the machine.[140]

One distinguishing characteristic of Still's osteopathy was that it united **biodynamics** with **biomechanics**. Nowadays it appears that some of his followers are separating this duality. Some osteopaths are pure "mechanics" and manipulate with more or less gentle techniques the entire organism, appreciating the laws of anatomy and physiology. They represent the biomechanical direction of osteopathy. In comparison, biodynamic practitioners place less emphasis on biomechanics but more on their sense of touch and the self-healing power of the organism. Similar to spiritual healers, they try to activate the self-healing power in the tissue, the only distinction being that they evaluate the rhythms of the organism diagnostically as well as therapeutically.[8, 9, 72]

In this context, a statement by Viola Frymann (training course, 2000) is relevant. She states that the **primary respiratory mechanism (PRM)** manifests clearly in healthy tissue. In the case of dysfunctions, however, the expressiveness of the PRM is disturbed, that is, observation of the PRM is useful in therapy as well as in diagnosis. Biodynamic practitioners take advantage of this phenomenon. With their hands, they create a fulcrum in the tissue.[8, 72, 135] After a certain time, the PRM manifests in different rhythms, which is an indication that the tissue is rediscovering its function.

Classical cranial osteopathy distinguishes itself from the biodynamic direction by the fact that it examines the tissue for movements and movement restrictions, with the purpose of then leading the structure to be treated back to a free motion direction and keeping the tissue there. As a result, the primary respiratory mechanism is able to unfold freely, without tensions, and hence to carry out the therapeutic effect.

The movements of the sphenobasilar synchondrosis (SBS; the mechanics of cranial motion) that Sutherland detected by sense of touch and then described, correspond to the movements of the head in the three spatial planes, including the sagittal plane (**up and down strain**) and horizontal plane (**lateral strain**). The functional techniques on the locomotor system follow the same principle. The therapist searches for a so-called balance point in all planes (**stacking**) and keeps the tissue in the relaxed position until an automatic release of tonicity occurs. We can see that the principles employed in cranial osteopathy are identical to those that apply to the rest of the body.

Opinions differ on the mechanism that is ultimately responsible for the release of tissue tension. Adherents of biomechanics posit that it is a reflective effect originating from the tissue receptors. Adherents of biodynamics believe in the effect of the PRM.

In his treatments, Still used a combination of so-called direct techniques with indirect techniques. Direct techniques manipulate the impaired segment in the corrective direction, while indirect techniques move the segment in the direction of the dysfunction.

While researching Still's method of treatment, Van Buskirk[23] asked older patients who had been treated by osteopaths in their childhood or youth, whether they could reconstruct the techniques they had been treated with. Some of these people were still able to describe the techniques, and much to his surprise Van Buskirk learned that these resembled the few techniques described by Still himself.

A short video clip still exists in which we can see Still treating a rib. This video, in combination with the statements by his patients and his limited writings indicates the following. After a thorough diagnosis, the therapist positions the impaired segment in the lesion position until the contracted musculature releases its tension. Then, the segment is moved into the corrected position under light pressure that is focused onto the blocked joint during the entire movement.

1.3   Scientific Evidence

As already mentioned, the nervous system played a central role for Still. It is the connecting link between the visceral, parietal, and cranial systems. Due to the research of Korr, Sato, Patterson, and others, the significance of the central nervous system and particularly the spinal cord in the formation of dysfunctions and pathologies has been scientifically proven.[79, 81, 112]

These scientists were able to explain experimentally the significance accorded to the spinal column by Still and other manual therapists in forming and maintaining pathologic states, and to confirm the central regulating role of the spinal cord. Korr[79] in particular succeeded in offering scientific explanations for generally accepted phenomena by experimentation. He referred to the locomotor system as "the primary machinery of life" and posited that the other systems (digestive, endocrine, and cardiovascular) are in its service.

In this context, the vegetative nervous system is particularly relevant. The two parts of the autonomous nervous system do not stand in an antagonistic, but in a complementary relationship. To put it simply, the parasympathetic division assists in the regeneration of the organism and also regulates longer-lasting processes. The sympathetic division, on the other hand, adapts the functions of the body's systems to immediate requirements. It intervenes in the regulation of blood supply to the active muscles, as, for example, by reducing the circulation of the digestive tract in favor of the musculature during physical activity. At the same time, it increases respiratory and pulse frequency and so on. The sympathetic division thus allows the organism to adapt spontaneously.

Korr provided neurophysiologic explanations for many phenomena that had been recognized by clinicians. He created the terms "**facilitated segment**" and "**neurologic lens.**" A facilitated segment is a segment of the spinal cord in which all nuclei have lower thresholds for irritation as a result of repeated stimulation or abnormal behavior of the segment due to chronic irritation. As a consequence, subliminal irritation suffices to stimulate the nuclei, and stimulation of facilitated segments often sets off a disproportionate reaction. An example is acute torticollis after exposure to a draft. The term "neurologic lens" refers to the following phenomenon: when a segment of the spinal cord is chronically irritated, it is susceptible to stimuli that should normally only irritate distant segments. This segment "attracts stimuli."

Korr's research team was able to provide additional interesting facts experimentally:

- Increasing the sympathetic tone (locally or in general) lowers the irritation threshold in the affected segments and increases muscle tone in those muscles that are supplied by these segments.
- Restricted motion in the spinal joints increases the sympathetic tone of segments and lowers the irritation threshold.
- Stress of all kinds increases muscle tone, especially in "facilitated segments."
- Postural imbalances affect the muscle tone in the paravertebral musculature and in the muscles supplied by the facilitated segments.
- Reducing the muscle tone of the paravertebral musculature lowers the sympathetic tone in these segments.

Two facts become evident from all these research findings:

- The musculoskeletal system is one of the key agencies for forming and maintaining somatic dysfunctions.
- The spinal cord has an important function as operator and organizer in the genesis of pathologic states.

Korr therefore did not exaggerate at all when he called the locomotor system the "primary machinery of life."

The myofascial structures play a key role in all important body functions, whether in breathing (thoracic as well as cellular respiration), circulation (diaphragm and muscles as venolymphatic pump), digestion (as mobilizer for the organs), or in the expression of emotions. The locomotor system facilitates motion, communication with others, food intake, and so on.

The fact that more than 80% of afferent nerves come from the locomotor system also speaks for the importance of the musculoskeletal system.[79, 112, 158] The extreme sensitivity of the muscle spindle (a pull of 1 g or stretch by 1 μm trigger a reaction in the muscle spindle)[79] makes the locomotor system an extremely sensitive organ. This facilitates fast reactions, but also makes it more susceptible to dysfunction. Contractions, malpostures, and disturbed coordination result.

Irvin (in [155]) and Kuchera[82] write that an inclination of 1–1.5 mm in the base of the sacrum suffices to change the muscle tone of the paravertebral musculature. Korr has described the resulting effects on the sympathetic nervous system and thereby on the entire organism. Nevertheless, the spinal cord as operational and organizational center is affected not only by peripheral stimulations.

A person's emotional state affects the genesis of dysfunctions and pathologies. In this context, the limbic system plays a decisive role.[158] As memory of the organism, it evaluates all stimuli and impressions as positive or negative for the person, depending on previous experiences. When a stimulus is received as pleasant, it gives positive feedback; if it is received as harmful, negative feedback results.

Via the hypothalamus–pituitary gland–adrenal gland axis, the neuroendocrinium is regulated, that is, the hormone balance as well as the neurovegetative system. Facilitated segments are affected particularly strongly by positive as well as negative emotional stimuli (see weekend migraines, stress ulcers). The segments with low irritation thresholds remain in a state of "chronic irritation" after a certain amount of time when subjected to continuous stimulation.[112] **To influence this state therapeutically, the complete lesion pattern must be treated to erase the impregnation of the pathologic pattern on the level of the CNS.** In this context, Korr referred to the spinal cord as "organizer of disease processes."[79]

The embryologically conditioned metamerism of the spinal cord results in a segmental unity between certain muscles, organs, vessels, areas of the skin, bones, and joints. Irritation in any one of these structures affects the functions of all the other structures associated with this segment.

Since neighboring segments are connected via interneurons, this facilitation generally applies to several segments. The plurisegmental supply of organs and muscles also supports this fact. In our opinion, it is wrong to associate an organ or function with a single segment of the spinal cord, especially since the brain does not recognize individual muscles but only motion patterns. In this context, congenital patterns and acquired patterns are equally significant.

In regard to the digestive system, it must be noted that it is subordinate to the functions of the organism as a whole in spite of its considerable autonomy through the enteric nervous system. The endocrinium and neurovegetative system also assume a regulating function here.

It is likely that acquired as well as congenital behavioral patterns are present here just as they are in the locomotor system. These patterns should correlate with those of the postural and locomotor systems and produce a certain type of person.[151]

1.4 Mobility and Stability

The locomotor system is composed of muscles and bones. It is supposed to fulfill two contrary functions simultaneously: on the one hand, it is supposed to provide stability, and, on the other, permit motion. The cerebellum and the organs of equilibrium make both of these functions possible. Both receive their information from receptors that are found primarily in myofascial structures.

The muscles are the executing organs for both of these functions: adequate basic muscle tone, quick responsiveness, and good coordination of muscle tension allow for graceful and harmonious movements as well as appropriate and subtle adjustments, to ensure balance with the least amount of effort.

Given how intelligent nature is, it has also solved this problem in a simple fashion. A centrifugal power (the expansive power of the organs) is controlled by an imploding power (the inherent tension of the muscles) in the musculature. The muscles' extraordinary sensitivity, in conjunction with precise coordination through the nervous system, facilitates an optimal, and therefore economical, stabilization of the locomotor system.

To execute harmonious movements, the muscles need a stable support, a central organ that coordinates the activity (the nervous system), and structures that guarantee supply (metabolism). The nervous system is responsible for the regulation of these activities. It activates agonists and synergists and inhibits antagonists exactly as needed to execute precise harmonious movements.

Most movement occurs unconsciously, with the involvement of a number of spinal reflexes. This is necessary for a person to act with foresight. The cerebrum requires decision-making freedom.

The spinal cord functions as operational center in all physical activities. Malfunctions can have disastrous results. All afferent nerves from the locomotor system reach the spinal cord, all efferent nerves to the muscles originate from here. Motion and postural patterns are carried here.

In the decade beginning in 1900, Sherrington described a series of reflex actions that explain these patterns (in [21] and in [160]). The muscles themselves consist of different muscle fibers with different properties. While the white (fast-twitch) fibers are good for fast contractions, the red (slow-twitch) fibers facilitate longer-lasting tension. Both have different pathologic tendencies. White fibers are prone to weakening and atrophy; the red ones to contracture and shortening. These properties must be taken into account during treatment.[40, 41, 86, 87]

1.5   The Organism as a Unit

As we already pointed out at the beginning of the introduction, the organism always reacts as a whole. We do not want to review the entire foundation of osteopathic theory here, but only those concepts that are necessary for understanding the following chapters.

Our organism *always* acts as a unit, in physiologic as well as pathologic states. The *entire* body participates in every physiologic process. Respiration, for example, involves all muscles, not only the respiratory muscles, the digestive muscles are mobilized according to a certain pattern, and circulation is supported by muscles.

This process also follows a set procedure. During inhalation, the entire locomotor system follows a motion pattern that Sutherland called "flexion–external rotation–abduction."[101, 102, 142, 143] Exhalation follows the reverse pattern: "extension–internal rotation–adduction."

Walking follows a similar pattern: the gait is also a harmonious series of movements in a consistent form and constantly recurring patterns from the tip of the big toe to the root of the nose. The holistic behavior of muscles is also found in pathologic conditions.

Human embryological development is the best evidence for holistic behavior: the fertilization of an ovum by a sperm results in division of the ovum into two cells with identical genetic code. This process of division continues until the cells combine into cell groups to form organs, muscles, bones, the nervous system, and so on. This common origin of all body cells suggests that all cells also react jointly to any given situation. The nervous system again appears to have a special function in this process as the control and coordination center.

Sutherland explains the unity of the human body by way of the membrane system and the fluctuation of liquor.[101, 102, 142, 143] When he speaks of **reciprocal tension membranes**, this refers to the fact that pulling on one base of the membrane system influences all other bases. The reciprocal tension membranes consist of the spinal and cranial dura mater.

Sutherland describes the following locations where the dural system attaches:
- Crista galli in front
- Clinoid process
- Pars petrosa left and right
- Inion in back
- Foramen magnum
- C2
- Sacrum

The practical consequence is that a change in the position of the sacrum, for example, automatically changes the position of the occipitoatlantoaxial (OAA) complex as well as of the cranial bones.

The dural system is filled with nerves and fluid (CSF) and continues via the nerve sheaths to the interstitium, which itself is also a fluid-filled space. In other words: changes in the dural system exert pressure on the fluids in the dural tube. These pressure changes spread through the entire interstitial fluid and thereby through the entire body.

According to Sutherland, the PRM, consisting of a flexion phase and an extension phase, causes pressure changes in the entire dural system and intercellular tissue, following a set rhythm in a tissue-specific direction and amplitude. The directions of movement correspond to those of thoracic respiration, that is, cranial flexion corresponding to inhalation, and cranial extension to exhalation.

Another proof of holism is found in the anatomy of the fasciae. Embryologically, the entire connective tissue originates from the mesoderm. The different layers are basically a single cover that divides the entire organism, covers organs and muscles, and constitutes the skin of the body. The three fascial layers of the body are interconnected. This continuity means that a change in one place, tension, or pressure, manifests throughout the entire tissue. This reciprocal property of the fasciae is what makes them so extraordinarily important for stasis, movement, and physical response to mechanical stress.[111] **The continuity of the fasciae, the continuity of the fluids, and the shared origin are signs of unity, in particular since all cells contain the same DNA.**

The entire body will always react as a unit, in physiology as in pathology. Any organ dysfunction will affect the muscles and joints that are segmentally connected to it. Due to the continuity of the myofascial tissue, the pull and pressure conditions in the *entire* organism and via the dural system in the cranium are changed. Stasis is adapted in a certain pattern, as is the cranium and the organs. The body strives to keep the functions of the entire organism undisturbed for as long as possible.

1.6 Interrelation of Structure and Function

All osteopaths are aware of the interrelation between structure and function. Just as structure stipulates function, function is dependent on structure. We can most easily explain this with the aid of the joint. To prevent it from stiffening, a joint has to remain movable. If its mobility is impaired, the joint membrane produces less fluid, the lack of strain and relief on the cartilage reduces its provision, and the joint capsule and cartilage become more brittle. This leads to reduced joint mobility to the point of arthritis or ankylosis. Arthritis is caused by malfunctioning of the joint, due to whatever causes.

The adaptation of structure to function is particularly evident in the locomotor system. Functional disturbances of the musculature result in structural changes. This process occurs surprisingly early,[2, 46] but fortunately is at least partially reversible. It takes about 30 days for functional disturbances to result in structural changes.[41, 82]

At the same time, structure stipulates function. Certain changes in the joints, for example, change the gait and disturb the normal function of other structures.

All osteopaths working in pediatrics are aware of the extent to which structure affects function. Still described the significance of osteopathic treatment for newborn infants.[140] Sutherland,[142, 143] Magoun,[101, 102] Frymann,[57] and Arbuckle[4] describe this subject in detail.

Structural changes at the cranial base in neonates due to pre- or perinatal complications are the source of functional disturbances in cranial nerves (X, XI, XII) and postural disturbances of the spinal column (scoliosis, kypholordosis). Magoun explains this by the craniosacral connection, and impaired growth by membranous tensions,[101] a theory that Korr[79] confirms.

Note: Still said exactly the same 50 years earlier when he claimed that disturbed circulation is the beginning of illness.[140] Herein, by circulation he meant both the venolymphatic as well as the arterial circulation and the circulation of nerve impulses. Structural changes are related to mechanical laws. Of significance are:

- Gravity
- Other external powers
- The form and condition of joint surfaces
- The influencing muscle pulls[107]

1.7 Biomechanics of the Spinal Column and the Locomotor System

Nobody has analyzed the biomechanics of the spinal column in as much detail as Littlejohn[53, 95, 96, 97, 98, 126] and Fryette[56] (among other aspects). While Littlejohn looks at the spinal column as a whole and tries to offer a mechanical explanation for common dysfunctions, Fryette describes the behavior of individual vertebrae in movements and in the case of certain dysfunctions. Littlejohn gives mechanical explanations for the behavior of the spinal column (globality).

The behavior of the spinal column and locomotor system in general is directed by mechanical laws. The spinal column, consisting of anteroposterior arches, and the joints, whose movements are dictated by ligaments, muscles, and joint surfaces, act under strain according to a specific pattern that then results in a corresponding adaptation by the rest of the locomotor system.

The spinal column consists of two anteriorly concave arches (thoracic spinal column [TSC] and sacrum) and two posteriorly concave arches (cervical spinal column [CSC] and lumbar spinal column [LSC]). Kypholordosis develops in the process of growing under the influence of powers affecting the body. Herein, congenital as well as acquired emotional factors should not be underestimated.[25, 86, 141] Perinatal microtraumas[4, 57, 102, 142, 143] and childhood traumas (falling onto the buttocks) can influence this process and cause scoliosis as well as increased kypholordosis.

Scoliosis commonly develops into s-shaped curvatures,[4, 82, 145] as if the entire spinal column made a rotation around a vertical axis in the horizontal plane. The horizontality of the base of the sacrum plays a key role in this process. An inclination of 1–1.5 mm in the frontal plane has a scoliosis-inducing effect on the spinal column. The extreme sensitivity of the muscle spindles is responsible for that.[82, 155]

It appears that the spinal column initially adjusts to a sudden inclination in the base of the sacrum with a global c-shaped scoliosis. However, postural factors activate the musculature to convert this into an s-shape as fast as possible. Littlejohn's model of the mechanics of the spinal column offers a mechanical explanation for this.[36, 96, 97] In addition to the anatomical circumstances of the joints, the muscles as executing organ are the key element in this adaptive process.

Scoliosis and kypholordosis not only affect the spinal column, but also the head, thorax, and extremities. The body as a whole participates in this process.[101]

The myofascial continuity, as well as the hydraulic system, consisting of the CSF and the interstitial fluid guarantee a holistic behavior. Structure adapts to function in a holistic fashion to ensure homeostasis.

1.8   The Significance of Homeostasis

Homeostasis is the maintenance of a relatively constant internal environment or of the organism's balance with the aid of regulatory cycles between the hypothalamus, the hormonal system, and the nervous system.[115] It serves to optimize all bodily functions for the sake of health. It is not a static condition, but a continually switching action between processes adapting to changing internal and external circumstances. Mechanical, electrophysiologic, and chemical processes regulate the bodily functions. Metabolism is ensured by pressure gradients, polarities, temperature differences, and drops in concentration.

The extracellular fluid is the environment in which these processes take place, and the connective tissue is the framework. The connective tissue plays a central role in homeostasis. Every cell participates in homeostasis and simultaneously profits from it.[111] This reciprocity makes the automatic regulation of all bodily functions possible.

When a dysfunction arises, the extracellular fluid reacts to correct the problem. If this does not succeed, increasingly more systems are affected. As a result, they are no longer able to contribute to homeostasis. This is the beginning of illness.

Changes in the myofascial tissue are the first indication for malfunctions because this is where the pathologic process takes place. Viscerosomatic reflexes induce changes in the myofascial structures, in particular in the paravertebral muscles, even in the case of minor organic disturbances.[111] This has been proven scientifically.[112] These neuromusculoskeletal reflexes are based on embryological connections. For therapy, it is significant that the body's self-healing power is able to restore homeostasis.

Somatovisceral reflexes, which have been documented by Sato (in [82, 112]), can be utilized therapeutically to influence organ dysfunctions. On the other hand, these reflexes highlight the extent of muscular imbalances and postural disturbances.

Paravertebral hypertonicity is not only an indication for segmental facilitation, but can also be its cause and thereby result in visceral disturbances. Besides injuries from accidents (sport- or work-related and so on) and asymmetrical physical activity, a difference in leg lengths is the most common reason for paravertebral hypertonicity.

1.9   The Nervous System as Control Center

The "primary machine of life"[79] is powered by muscles. **The musculature is the organ of the locomotor system, and the nervous system is the control center**. To carry out harmonious movements, the muscles have to cooperate with each other. They do this by working in chains, wherein one unit of movement gives support to the next one.

Example: To allow the biceps brachii to flex the elbow, the shoulder has to be prevented from being pulled forward. This is ensured by the extensors of the shoulder and the stabilizers of the scapula. In

this way, loop-shaped chains are formed, so-called lemniscates. Because most muscles run diagonally or are fan-shaped in structure, the lemnisci occur in the sagittal as well as in the frontal plane.

The nervous system recruits muscles for motion processes. Congenital reflexes make this job easier for the organism. Receptors in the muscles, tendons, fasciae, and joint system deliver information on movements and in conjunction with the centers of postural and directed motility, facilitate finely coordinated movements and adequate adjustments to changes in balance.

1.10   Different Models of Muscle Chains

Several models for myofascial chains exist (see Chapter 8). Rolfers, physiotherapists, and osteopaths have all described muscle chains. These chains differ from each other not only because opinions vary, but also because of different therapeutic emphasis. A Rolfer does not focus on the same things in treatment as an osteopath or a physiotherapist.

The model that we present in Chapter 8 is based on Sutherland's theory of two motion patterns:
• Flexion–abduction–exterior rotation
• Extension–adduction–interior rotation

Sutherland did not describe muscle chains as such, but the behavior of segments in both of these patterns. An interesting fact of his model is that it corresponds to the motions of respiration and gait.

Because we take the holistic principle as our basis in physiology and pathology, we are convinced that cranial patterns continue in the locomotor system as in the visceral area and vice versa. The factors described above (fluids, membranes, continuity of the connective tissue) guarantee this. In addition, physical and mechanical laws ensure that the joints of the entire locomotor system (including the cranial sutures) carry this pattern into the entire musculoskeletal system. This holds true regardless of whether the trigger of the pattern is a vertebra, the ilium, an organ, or a cranial bone.

The entire organism adjusts to dysfunctional or pathogenic elements so that the body can function as optimally and painlessly as possible. This reduces tensions, harmonizes pressure conditions, and maintains circulation.

All this is needed to allow the body's self-healing powers to carry out their work. According to cranial osteopathic theory, this sustains the primary respiratory mechanism, through which the "breath of life" reaches the cells.

1.11 In This Book

In the first part of this book (Part A), we introduce several models of myofascial chains (Chapter 2) before laying out the physiologic foundations for the behavior of the locomotor system (Chapter 3).

In the next section (Chapter 4), we present Sutherland's cranial concept, limiting ourselves to the biomechanical aspect. We describe the physiologic motions of the sphenobasilar synchondrosis (SBS) and the effects on the spinal column and the locomotor system. The locus of the sacrum depends on the position of the occiput above the atlas. This in turn determines the position of the spinal column, extremities, and thorax.

Chapter 5 deals with the mechanics of the spinal column as seen by Littlejohn. Littlejohn's theory is a functional model, rooted in clinical practice. It explains the behavior of individual spinal column segments towards each other. The SAT model (specific adjusting technique) that was developed by Bradbury and elaborated by Dummer[51, 52, 53] is a logical and clinically extremely valuable application of Littlejohn's model.

In the next section (Chapter 6), we introduce a number of interesting discoveries and ideas by Janda, which are primarily of clinical relevance. Chapter 7 deals with a very simple rational form of diagnosis: the Zink patterns. This refers to an examination of the myofascial torsion patterns at the junctions of the spinal column. We use this model to detect the dominant region (see Practical Application part of the chapter). In the same chapter, we also compare the models of Littlejohn and Zink, and the neurophysiologic and anatomical factors. We find that Zink and Littlejohn's models can be projected onto each other and that there are neurophysiologic connections that help to explain these findings. This emphasizes the functional and structural interrelations.

In Chapter 8, we introduce a model of muscle chains that is based on Sutherland's two patterns. We describe the behavior of the different motion units of the body and the formation of kypholordosis and scoliosis and the affected muscles. This model differs from the other models in a number of essential points.

We believe that the various motion units act like cogwheels, similar to the behavior of the cranial bones in Sutherland's craniosacral model. In this process, movements in opposite directions between two consecutive motion units occur. This explains kypholordosis and scoliosis, as well as opposing rotations between units (see foot, knee, and hip positions in knock or bow legs).

We see the **flexors** as the muscles in the concavities of the locomotor system, and the **extensors** as the muscles in its convexities. A dominance of flexor chains thus automatically causes an increase in curvature, and a dominance of extensor chains a stretching of the skeleton. Because the organism consists of two equal halves embryologically, each body half has one flexor chain and one extensor chain. The nervous system directs the coordination between the two sides.

In this part of the book, we describe the muscle chains and explain the formation of posture disturbances. Here we want to emphasize that our model does not lay claim to completeness but is merely an attempt to explain phenomena observed in daily clinical practice. Intensive research in the literature of the field and attendance of seminars have answered many of our questions and finally led us to write a book on this interesting topic.

The second part of the book (Part B) is concerned with practice. Here we present a diagnostic model and describe a few treatment methods. For examination, we rely on the "Zink patterns" (see Chapter 7) and on simple traction tests, on the basis of which we can find the dominant structure extremely quickly. We limit our discussion here to the treatment of myofascial structures. It is self-evident that organic disturbances and cranial dysfunctions must be treated with adequate treatment methods. In this part of the book, we also present in detail the diagnosis and treatment of trigger points. This is a form of therapy that provides very fast sedation of pain for acute as well as chronic complaints and returns the structural changes in the myofascial unit back to normalcy.

2 Models of Myofascial Chains

2.1 Herman Kabat 1950: Proprioceptive Neuromuscular Facilitation

Dr. Herman Kabat founded the proprioceptive neuro-muscular facilitation (PNF) concept in the 1940s. He developed this treatment method originally for the treatment of poliomyelitis patients. Kabat was supported by Margaret Knott and Dorothy Voss, who published the first book on PNF in 1956. Since then, the method has been refined and successfully applied in patients with other symptoms.

The concept of PNF is based on the neurophysiologic findings of Sir Charles Sherrington[21, 160]:
- Reciprocal innervation or inhibition
- Spatial summation
- Spread of the stimulus response (temporal summation)
- Successive temporary summation (successive induction)
- Irradiation (irritability)
- Postisometric relaxation (PIR) (after discharge)

Kabat developed a treatment technique wherein weak muscles are integrated into a muscle chain. The muscle chain is stimulated with the aid of specific stimuli (by visual, auditive, and tactile irritants). This process takes optimal advantage of the nerve and muscle properties described by Sherrington, in order to integrate optimally the weak muscle (or muscle group) into the motion pattern.

The proprioceptive capabilities of the locomotor system are stimulated to strengthen weak muscles and to coordinate motion processes. The intention is to give the central nervous system positive inputs and thereby facilitate normal motion patterns via central regulatory cycles. Therefore, the same motion patterns are applied continuously.

▪ Motion Patterns

The following motion patterns are stimulated:

For the Scapula and Pelvis
- Anterior elevation
- Anterior depression
- Posterior elevation
- Posterior depression

For the Upper Extremity
- Flexion–abduction–external rotation
- Extension–adduction–internal rotation
- Flexion–adduction–external rotation
- Extension–abduction–internal rotation

For the Lower Extremity
- Flexion–abduction–internal rotation
- Extension–adduction–external rotation
- Flexion–adduction–external rotation
- Extension–abduction–internal rotation

For the Neck
- Leftward flexion–rightward extension and vice versa
- Flexion–lateral leftward flexion–leftward rotation and vice versa
- Extension–lateral rightward flexion–rightward rotation and vice versa

For the Torso
- Trunk flexion–lateral flexion–leftward (or rightward) rotation
- Trunk extension–lateral flexion–rightward (or leftward) rotation

Regarding the extremity patterns, the motion directions above refer to the large joints adjacent to the trunk, namely the shoulder and hip. Two antagonistic motion patterns form a diagonal.

◾ Application Modalities

- The starting position of the patient can vary (supine, prone, lateral, sitting, standing).
- The segment to be treated is pre-stretched in such a way that all muscles involved in the pattern (agonists and synergists) are stretched.
- Pre-stretching as well executing the motions should be painless.
- Evasive motions are corrected.
- The therapist asks the patient to move in the desired direction and stimulates this direction by tactile contact or resistance.
- In the end position of the movement, the agonists and synergists of the motion pattern are optimally shortened while their antagonists are stretched.
- The movement generally begins in the distal joints of the segment and progresses continuously to the proximal joints.
- Special attention is paid to the rotational component because it is significant for the pattern.
- The intermediary joints (elbow or knee) can remain or be stretched or bent as needed during the movement. The proximal joints (shoulder and hip) and the distal joints, however, carry out identical movements.
- Patterns can be combined.
- The various Sherrington principles are taken into consideration.

◾ Observations

1. Kabat emphasizes muscle chain movements, not movement components of individual muscles.
2. Similar to the way in which Sherrington treats the nervous system as a unit, Kabat views the musculature as a unit.
3. Kabat describes different patterns for the upper extremity and the lower extremity.
4. In the patterns of the upper extremities, flexion and external rotation are associated, and extension and internal rotation.
5. In the patterns of the lower extremities, abduction (ABD) and internal rotation, and adduction and external rotation go together.

2.2 Godelieve Struyff-Denys

Godelieve Struyff-Denys, a Belgian physiotherapist with osteopathic training (European School of Osteopathy, Maidston, Kent) was apparently the first to speak of muscle chains in the true sense of the word.[141] She was familiar with Kabat's principle of PNF, as well as with Mézière's spinal column therapy. In addition, her work was clearly influenced by Piret and Béziers, who stressed that a movement depends on the shape of the joint surfaces and the disposition of the musculature, especially of the pluriarticular muscles.

According to Piret and Béziers, these two factors lead to spiral-shaped motions. As a result, tonicity arises that gives the segment its form and structure (S. Piret and M.M. Béziers: *La Coordination Motrice*, Masson 1971). In other words: the shape of the body is conditioned by motion patterns that in turn reflect the person's emotional state. This reveals the psychological component that Ms. Struyff-Denis valued so highly.

The Mézière method consists of a restructuring of the locomotor system. Impaired coordination of the myoskeletal system is taken as the cause of postural defects. The psyche is irrelevant for Mézière. The innovative aspect of this method at that time (1960s) was that it broke with the traditional treatment of the spinal column, according to which it was straightened by strengthening the dorsal muscles.

For Mézière, kyphosis, lordosis, and scoliosis are not the result of muscular insufficiency, but of tonicity in the dorsal muscle chain. Additionally, a hypertonic dorsal muscle chain is the cause of weakened abdominal muscles and of impaired coordination. Treatment can therefore only aim at reducing tonicity in the dorsal muscle chain from head to foot.

Struyff-Denys adapted the principle of muscle chains from Kabat, and the principle of treatment by stretching from Mézière. Piret and Béziers added the psychological dimension. From these foundations grew the first holistic model of muscle chains.

Struyff-Denys describes 10 muscle chains, five in each half of the body. These chains normally function in a coordinated fashion to execute spiral-shaped movements. In most of these, one of the myofascial chains dominates. The dominant chain gives the organism its shape and the person their specific gestures. Struyff-Denis never doubted that it was impossible to neutralize the dominant chain entirely. This would have been comparable to changing the type of person they were completely. The most we can do is to create balance in an overly dominant chain to facilitate coordinated movements and prevent deformations.

Muscular imbalance can arise from three causes. For Struyff-Denis, they are the following:

1. The key cause is the psyche: a person's posture, gesture, and morphology are primarily a reflection of their psychological condition.
2. The second cause is lifestyle: work habits, sports, but also lack of movement cause false muscle strain and uneven muscle tone.
3. The third factor also influences the myofascial structures via central regulatory cycles. Stress, anger, worrying, sorrow, and other emotional factors are able to affect the tone of certain muscle chains temporarily or permanently.

■ Classification of the Five Muscle Chains

The five muscle chains of each half of the body are composed as follows:

- Three fundamental or vertical muscle chains involving the head and trunk.
- Two complementary or horizontal chains that concern the upper and lower extremities. These are relational chains that relate the person to their surroundings.

These five muscle chains correspond to five psychological constitutions that are likewise categorized into three fundamental and two complementary constitutions.

Interestingly, Struyff-Denys assigned to each of the vertical fundamental chains a region of the cranium. The shape (forward bulge, flattening and so on) of this cranial region is an indication of the dominance of a certain psychological constitution. The vertical chains have muscular extensions into the extremities, just as the horizontal muscle chains are connected by torso muscles with the axial skeleton and thereby with the vertical chains.

Following is a list of the muscle sections of the five muscle chains. For further information, the reader should refer to the original source.[40]

The Vertical or Fundamental Muscle Chains

The Anteromedian Chain (Fig. 2.1)

Primary Section: Ventral Torso Muscles
- Pelvic floor muscles
- Rectus abdominis
- Lower and median sections of the pectoralis major
- Transversus thoracis
- Intercostal muscles (median section)
- Subclavius
- Scalenus anterior
- Sternal section of the sternocleidomastoideus (SCM)
- Hyoid muscles

Secondary Section: Lower Extremity
- Pyramidalis abdominis
- Adductors
- Gracilis
- Median section of the gastrocnemius
- Adductor hallucis longus

Upper Extremity
- Anterior section of the deltoideus
- Brachialis
- Supinator
- Abductors pollicis

The Posteromedian Chain (Fig. 2.2)
Primary Section
- Erector trunci muscles
- Long nuchal extensors

Secondary Section: Lower Extremity
- Semimembranosus
- Semitendinosus
- Soleus
- Toe flexors

Upper Extremity
- Latissimus dorsi
- Pars ascendens of the trapezius
- Infraspinatus
- Teres minor
- Back section of the deltoideus
- Long section of the triceps brachii
- Finger flexors
- Pronators

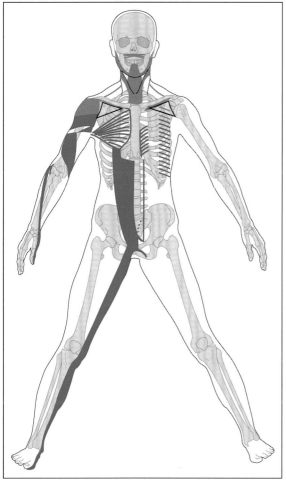

Fig. 2.1 Anteromedian chain according to Struyff-Denys.

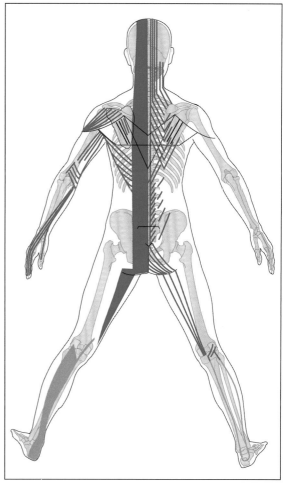

Fig. 2.2 Posteromedian chain according to Struyff-Denys.

The Posteroanterior–Anteroposterior Chain (Fig. 2.3)

Primary Section
- Autochthonous or deep paravertebral muscles
- Respiratory muscles
- Splenius capitis and colli
- Scalenus
- Iliopsoas

Secondary Section: Lower Extremity
- Vastus medialis
- Rectus femoris
- Toe extensors

Upper Extremity
- Pectoralis minor
- Coracobrachialis
- Short section of the biceps brachii
- Median section of the triceps brachii
- Finger extensors

The Horizontal or Complementary Muscle Chains

The Posterolateral Chain (Fig. 2.4)

Lower Extremity
- Gluteus medius
- Biceps femoris
- Vastus externus
- Peronei muscles
- Gastrocnemius lateralis
- Plantaris
- Lateral section of the abductor

Upper Extremity
- Pars horizontalis and descendens of the trapezius
- Supraspinatus
- Median section of the deltoideus
- Lateral part of the triceps brachii
- Anconeus
- Extensor carpi ulnari
- Flexor carpi ulnari
- Abductor digiti minimi

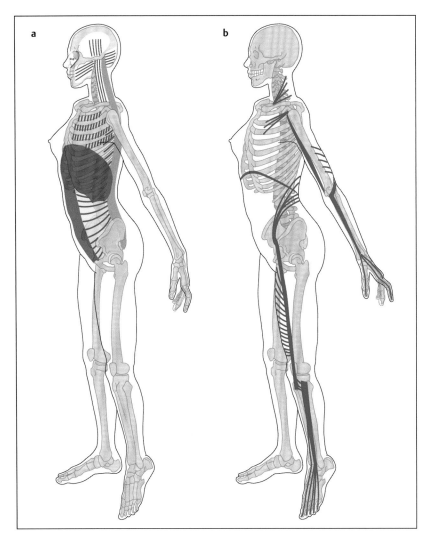

Fig. 2.3a, b Posteroanterior–anteroposterior chain according to Struyff-Denys.

The Anterolateral Chain (Fig. 2.5)

Lower Extremity

- Gluteus medius
- Tensor fasciae latae (TFL)
- Tibialis anterior
- Tibialis posterior
- Interossei plantaris muscles
- Lumbricalis muscles

Upper Extremity

- Pars clavicularis of the SCM, pectoralis minor, and deltoideus muscles:
- Teres major
- Latissimus dorsi
- Subscapularis
- Long part of the biceps brachii
- Superficial part of the supinator
- Brachioradialis
- Extensor carpi radialis longus and brevis
- Palmaris longus
- Thenar muscles
- Lumbricales and interossei palmaris muscles
- Flexor carpi radialis

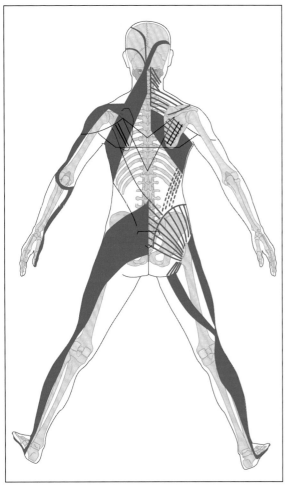

Fig. 2.4 Posterolateral chain according to Struyff-Denys.

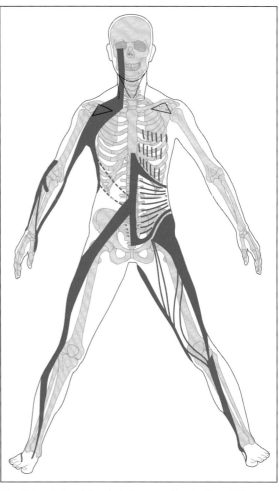

Fig. 2.5 Anterolateral chain according to Struyff-Denys.

2.3 Thomas W. Myers

■ "Anatomy Trains"—Myofascial Meridians (Chains)

Tom Myers, certified Rolfer and docent at the Rolf Institute, describes a series of myofascial chains in the technical terminology of Rolfers in his book *Anatomy Trains*.[108] For presenting the chains, he employs metaphors like tracks, platforms, express trains, and so on. Thereby, the rather complex chains are brought into a tangible, plastic form.

The myofascial connections are presented in a simple and comprehensible manner. Holism and myofascial continuity dominate. Fascial trains continue throughout the entire body, with the train lines (or myofascial meridians) going in the same direction. Osseous attachments of muscles or fasciae comprise so-called relay stations (train stations) and thereby acquire special significance.

The myofascial meridians allow for an analysis based on whole-body posture and thereby allow the informed therapist to treat the shortened meridians specifically.

Myers describes seven myofascial meridians or chains, which we will present here only briefly.

■ Myofascial Chains According to T. Myers

The Superficial Back Line (Fig. 2.6)

- Fascia plantaris
- Triceps surae
- Ischiocrural muscles
- Sacrotuberal ligament

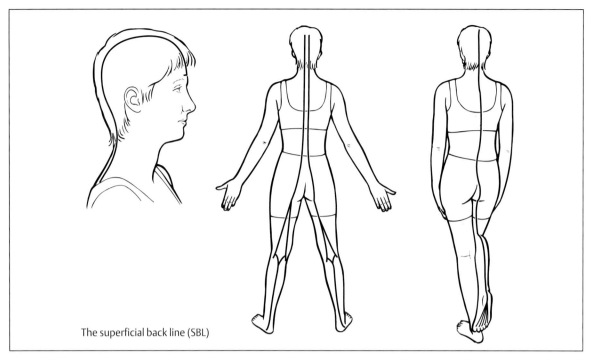

The superficial back line (SBL)

Fig. 2.6 Myofascial chains according to Myers. Superficial back line.

- Erector spinae muscles
- Suboccipital muscles
- Galea aponeurotica

The Superficial Front Line (Fig. 2.7a)

- Anterior compartment muscles
- Infrapatellar and quadriceps tendons
- Rectus abdominis
- Sternalis and pectoralis major
- SCM

The Lateral Line (Fig. 2.7b)

- Sole of the foot and peroneal muscle
- Tractus iliotibialis, TFL, and gluteus maximus
- Obliquii and quadratus lumborum muscles
- Intercostal muscle
- Splenius and SCM

The Spiral Line (Fig. 2.7c–e)

- Splenius capitis
- Rhomboideus and serratus anterior on the other side
- Obliquii muscles
- TFL and tractus iliotibialis
- Tibialis anterior
- Peroneus longus
- Biceps femoris
- Sacrotuberal ligament
- Erector spinae back to the starting point

This line encircles the thorax and induces torsion in the chest.

The Arm Lines

There are four arm lines (**Fig. 2.8**), one on each side of each arm, from the thorax or occiput up to the fingers:
- Deep front arm line
- Superficial front arm line
- Deep back arm line
- Superficial back arm line

The Functional Lines

The functional lines are diagonal extensions of the arm lines to the pelvis on the opposite side. They connect the two sides of the body with each other:
- Functional back line
- Functional front line

The Deep Front Line

- Sole of the foot
- Dorsal compartment muscles
- Hip adductors
- Iliopsoas

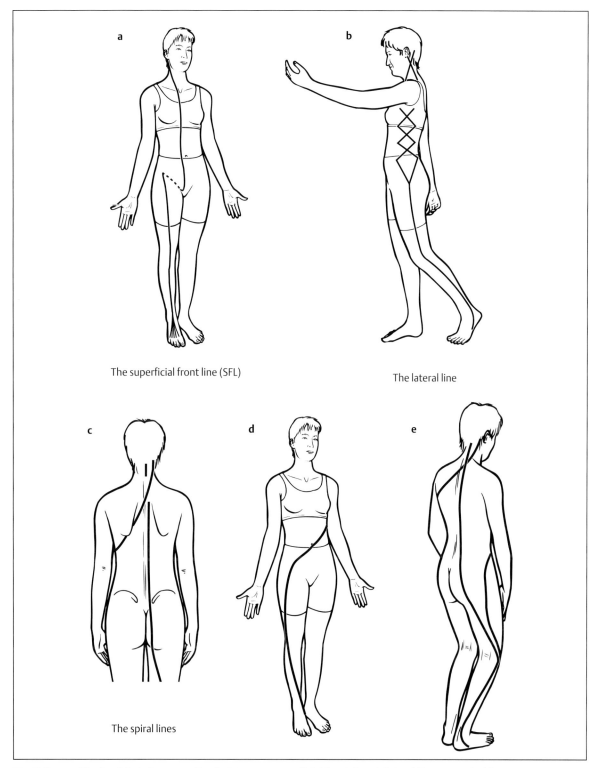

a

The superficial front line (SFL)

b

The lateral line

c

The spiral lines

d

e

Fig. 2.7a–e Myofascial chains according to Myers: **a** superficial front line, **b** lateral line, **c–e** spiral lines.

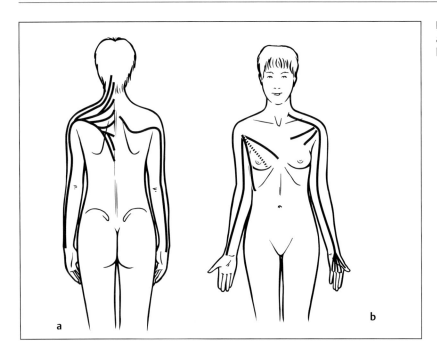

Fig. 2.8a, b Myofascial chains according to Myers: **a** back arm lines, **b** frontal arm lines.

- Anterior longitudinal ligament
- Diaphragms
- Mediastinum with pericard
- Pleura
- Scaleni muscles
- Hyoid muscles
- Muscles of mastication

In spite of the fact that these chains are very theoretical and not always easily comprehensible, they provide an explanation for the manifestation of symptoms.

2.4 Leopold Busquet

■ The Muscle Chains

The French osteopath, Leopold Busquet, produced an entire book series on the topic of muscle chains .[25–30] The first four volumes describe the muscle chains of the trunk and extremities. The fifth volume deals with the cranial connections of the torso muscle chains. The last book of the series describes the visceral connections of the abdominal organs via the suspension system (mesenteries, ligaments, omenta) and the peritoneum to the trunk.

In addition, Leopold Busquet wrote two further books about cranial osteopathy[24, 29a]. We should note that some of his statements contradict what Sutherland and the other Anglo-American cranial experts say. For example, he describes the palpatory signs of cranial torsion and sidebending rotation contrary to Sutherland (in [102]).

Of interest are the connections that Busquet draws between organ dysfunctions (and pathologies) and posture. The author describes two groups of organ dysfunctions and their respective effects on the locomotor system:

- Expansive organic disturbances (e.g., liver stasis) that force the muscles to make the necessary space for the organ (**Fig. 2.9**)
- Retractive or painful processes in which the muscles are recruited to provide better support for the organ or to slacken the sore tissue and thereby lower pain (antalgic posture in abdominal inflammation) (**Fig. 2.10**)

Leopold Busquet   **19**

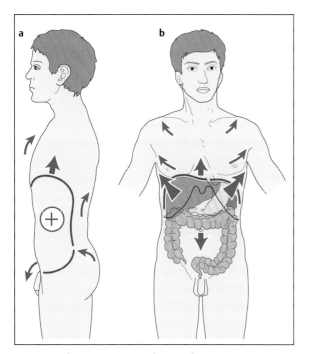

Fig. 2.9a, b "Opening tendency" during expansive processes in the abdomen.

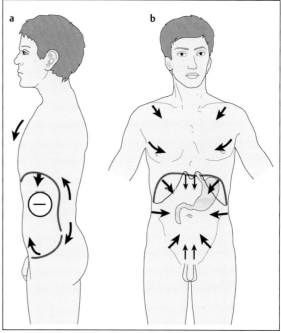

Fig. 2.10a, b "Closing tendency" (curling in) during support-seeking processes and spasms in the abdomen.

Visceral disturbances can cause postural malpositions like scoliosis, kypholordosis, flat and high arched foot, as well as the starting point for muscle, tendon, or joint injuries.

◼ Myofascial Chains According to Busquet

Busquet describes five chains on the trunk that run into the extremities:
- Static posterior chain
- Flexion chain or straight anterior chain
- Extension chain or straight posterior chain
- Diagonal posterior chain or "opening chain"
- Diagonal anterior chain or "closing chain"

The Static Posterior Chain (Fig. 2.11)

When standing, gravity tends to top the upper body forward. The body counteracts this with two passive (that is, using little energy) mechanisms. These are, on the one hand, the pleural and peritoneal spaces that exert an expansive power and, on the other hand, a ligamentous and fascial chain from the frontal bone to the sacrum.

Fig. 2.11a, b Static posterior chain according to Busquet.

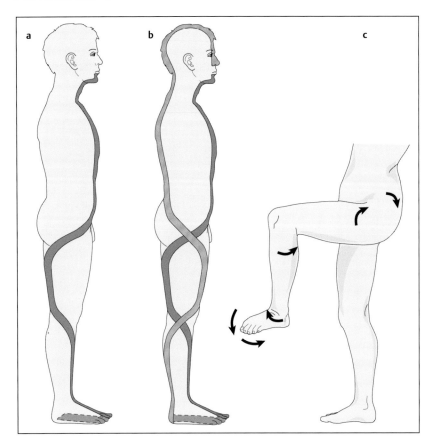

Fig. 2.12a–c   Flexion chain, or straight anterior chain, according to Busquet.

On the other extremities, it continues on the outside of the legs all the way to the feet. This is for good reason: during walking, gravity tends to tip the body weight toward the leg in the swinging phase.

Note: An alternative explanation for these facts is offered by evolutionary history. In the course of evolution, an internal rotation of the lower (back) extremities occurred, which caused the dorsal muscles of the leg to be positioned laterally. As part of this process, the knees and feet shifted so that their motion plane was oriented toward the locomotion plane. As a result, the dorsal structures of the leg shifted outward. Hence, evolutionary history demonstrates here how structure adapted to function. The static posterior chain consists of the following structures, from cranial to caudal positions:

- Falx cerebri and cerebelli
- Ligaments of the vertebral arch
- Thoracolumbar fascia
- Sacrotuberal and spinal ligament
- Fascia of the piriformis and obturator muscles
- Tensor fasciae latae
- Fibula and interosseous membrane
- Plantar fascia

Flexion Chain or Straight Anterior Chain (Fig. 2.12)

Busquet assigns the following roles to this chain:
- Flexion
- Global kyphosis of the trunk
- Physical and psychological "curling up"
- Introversion

It is composed of the following muscles:

On the Trunk

- The anterior intercostal muscles
- Rectus abdominis
- Pelvic floor muscles

Connection to the Shoulder Blade

- Transversus thoracis
- Pectoralis minor
- Pars descendens of the trapezius (connects to the spinal column)

Connection to the Upper Arm

- Pectoralis major
- Teres major
- Rhomboidei

Connection to the Cervical Spine
- Scaleni
- Splenius colli

Connection to the Head
- Subclavius
- SCM
- Splenius capitis

Connection to the Lower Extremity
- Iliopsoas

On the Upper Extremity

According to Busquet, the upper extremity does not follow the standard reversal between flexion and extension. The flexor chains of the upper extremity hence consist of the anterior muscles:
- Anterior part of the deltoideus
- Coracobrachialis
- Biceps brachialis
- Brachialis
- Hand and finger flexors

On the Lower Extremity

The following movements result from an activation of the flexor chain in the leg:
- Backward rotation of the ilium
- Hip flexion
- Knee flexion
- Dorsal extension in the ankle joint
- Increase of the foot arch

The flexor chain of the leg consists of the following muscles:

Backward Rotation of the Ilium
- Rectus abdominis
- Psoas minor
- Semimembranosus

Hip Flexion
- Iliopsoas
- Internal and external obturators

Knee Flexion
- Semimembranosus
- Popliteus

Dorsal Extension of the Foot
- Extensor digitorum longus

Plantar Flexion of the Toes and Increase of the Foot Arch
- Quadratus plantae
- Flexor hallucis brevis

- Flexor digiti minimi brevis
- Lumbricales

Extension Chain or Straight Posterior Chain (Fig. 2.13)

The extension chain has the following functions:
- Extension
- Global lordosis of the trunk
- Opening outward
- Communicating with the surroundings

It is composed of the following elements:

On the Trunk
Deep Plane
- Autochthonous muscles
- Erector trunci
- Iliocostal part of the quadratus lumborum

Median Plane
- Superior and inferior posterior serratus muscles

Connection to the Shoulder Blade
- Pars horizontalis and descendens of the trapezius
- Pectoralis minor
- Transverses thoracis

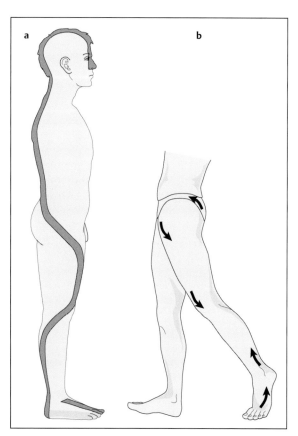

Fig. 2.13a, b Extension chain, or straight posterior chain, according to Busquet.

Connection to the Arm
- Latissimus dorsi
- Teres major
- Pectoralis major

Connection to the Cervical Spine
- Splenius colli
- Scaleni
- Spinotransversal paravertebral muscles

Connection to the Head
- Splenius capitis
- Pars ascendens of the trapezius
- SCM

Connection to the Lower Extremity
- Gluteus maximus

On the Upper Extremity

The extensors of the upper extremity are the posterior muscles:
- Posterior part of the deltoideus
- Triceps brachii
- Hand and finger extensors

On the Lower Extremity

The extensor chain turns the ilium forward, extends the hip and knee, makes a plantar flexion in the ankle joint, and lowers the foot arch.

Ilium Rotation Forward
- Quadratus lumborum
- Rectus femoris

Hip Extension
- Gluteus maximus
- Quadratus femoris

Knee Extension
- Vastus intermedius of the quadriceps
- Plantar flexion of the foot
- Plantaris

Extension of the Forefoot
- Flexor digitorum brevis

Extension of the Toes
- Interossei muscles
- Extensor digitorum brevis
- Extensor hallucis brevis

The Diagonal Posterior Chain or "Opening Chain" (Fig. 2.14)

The diagonal chains facilitate torsion of the trunk. The anterior diagonal chains cause a forward torsion, and the posterior ones a backward torsion. When both ventral diagonal chains dominate, the shoulders and both iliac bones are pulled forward medially. Both dorsal diagonal chains pull the shoulders and iliac bones backward. In the lower extremities, they have a similar effect.

The dorsal diagonal chains cause abduction and external rotation in the leg, while the anterior diagonal chains cause adduction and internal rotation of the legs.

Composition of the posterior diagonal chain:

> Note: Busquet names the diagonal chains according to their origin at the ilium. The right diagonal chain connects the right ilium to the left shoulder!

Right Diagonal Opening Chain

On the Trunk
- Iliolumbar fibers of the right paravertebral muscles
- Iliolumbar fibers of the right quadratus lumborum
- Iliocostal fibers of the left quadratus lumborum
- Left internal intercostal muscles
- Left inferior posterior serratus

Connection to the Left Shoulder
- Pars ascendens of the left trapezius
- Left pectoralis minor
- Left transversus thoracis

Connection to the Left Arm
- Left latissimus dorsi
- Left teres major
- Left pectoralis major

Connection to the Cervical Spine
- Left splenius colli
- Left scaleni muscles

Connection to the Head
- Left splenius capitis
- Left SCM
- Left trapezius

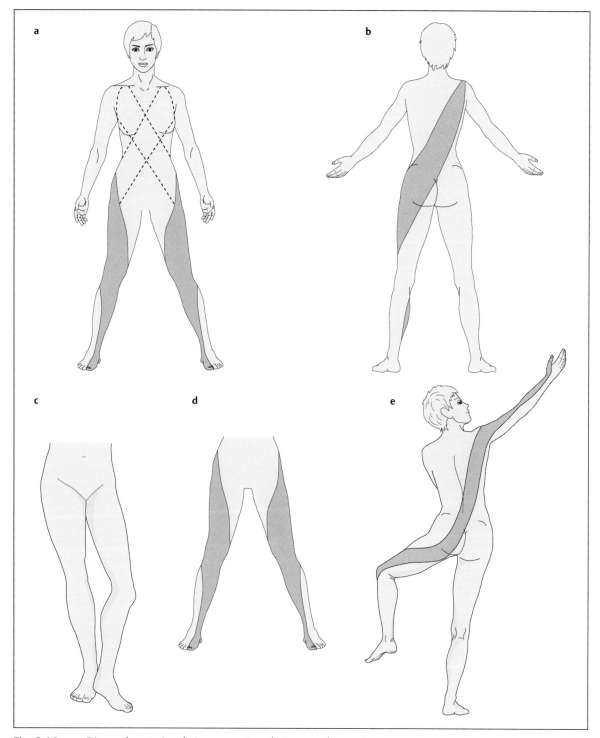

Fig. 2.14a–e Diagonal posterior chain, or opening chain, according to Busquet.

Connection to the Right Leg
• Superficial part of the gluteus maximus

In this chain, the ilium makes an outflare, the hip an ABD and external rotation, the knee a varus position, the foot a supination.

The following muscles of the lower extremity are involved:

Outflare of the Ilium
• Levator ani
• Ischiococcygeus
• Sartorius
• TFL
• Gluteal muscles

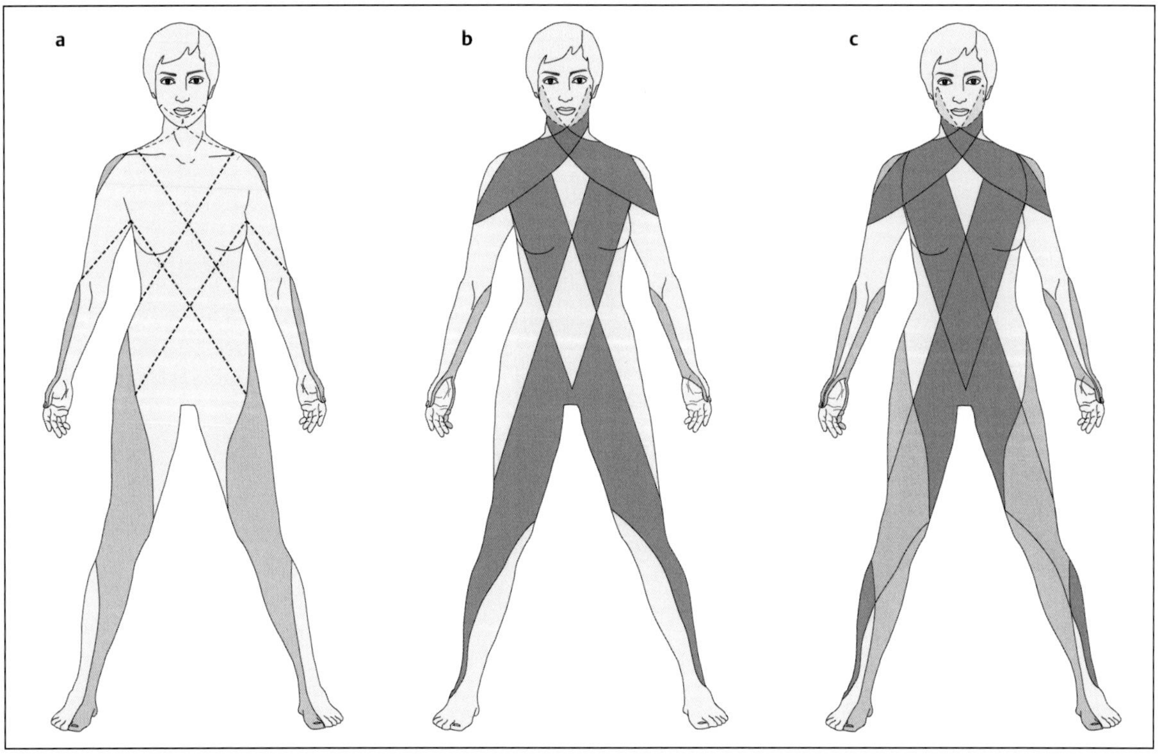

Fig. 2.15a–c   Diagonal anterior chain, or closing chain, according to Busquet.

Abduction and Outward Rotation of the Hip
- Piriformis
- Gluteus maximus and medius

Outward Rotation and Varus of the Knee
- Biceps femoris
- Vastus lateralis

Varus of the Hindfoot and Supination
- Anterior tibialis
- Posterior tibialis
- Extensor hallucis longus

Diagonal Anterior Chain or "Closing Chain"
(Fig. 2.15)

The left diagonal anterior chain serves as an example here (left ilium to right shoulder).

On the Trunk
- Deep plane: left obliquus internus
- Superficial plane: right obliquus externus
- Right external intercostal muscles
- Right posterior superior serratus

Connection to the Right Shoulder
- Right transversus thoracis
- Right pectoralis minor
- Pars ascendens of the right trapezius

- Right anterior serratus
- Right rhomboidei

Connection to the Right Arm
- Right pectoralis major
- Right teres major
- Right rhomboidei

Connection to the Cervical Spine
- Right scaleni muscles
- Left splenius colli

Connection to the Head
- Right subclavius
- Right SCM
- Left splenius capitis
- Pars descendens of the left trapezius

Connection to the Lower Extremity
- Pyramidalis abdominis

Dominance of this muscle chain results in an inflare of the ilium, internal rotation and abduction of the hip, valgus of the knee and hindfoot, pronation of the foot, and bunion. The involved muscles are:
- Inflare of the ilium: obliquus internus
- Adduction and internal rotation of the femur: abductors, pectineus

- Inward rotation of the tibia: gracilis, semitendinosus, medial vastus
- Valgus of the knee: lateral gastrocnemius
- Valgus of the calcaneus and pronation of the foot: peronei muscles, abductor digiti minimi, abductor hallucis longus

■ Functions of the Myofascial Muscle Chains

- The five muscle chains are responsible for all movements of the trunk.
- The two anterior straight chains cause flexion.
- The two posterior straight chains cause extension.
- The right anterior and posterior straight chains cause a rightward inclination.
- The left anterior and posterior straight chains cause a leftward inclination.

- The left anterior diagonal chain causes a left anterior trunk torsion.
- The right anterior diagonal chain causes a right anterior trunk torsion.
- The left posterior diagonal chain causes a left posterior trunk torsion.
- The right posterior diagonal chain causes a right posterior trunk torsion.
- The right anterior diagonal chain and the left posterior diagonal chain cause a rightward rotation of the trunk.
- The left anterior diagonal chain and the right posterior diagonal chain cause a leftward rotation of the trunk.
- The left anterior and the left posterior diagonal chain cause a left translation.
- The two anterior diagonal chains "close the body."
- The two posterior diagonal chains "open the body."

2.5 Paul Chauffour: Le Lien Mécanique en Osteopathie (The Mechanical Link in Osteopathy)

■ Paul Chauffour's Biomechanical Chains

In his book *Le Lien Mécanique Ostéopathique,*[45] the French osteopath Paul Chauffour, with J.M. Guillot, clearly describes the topography of the fasciae, the places where they attach to the skeleton, and their functions. Furthermore, the chapter on "Osteofascial Biomechanics" (Biomécanique Ostéo-faciale) presents the myofascial chains in the four main movements of the body:
- Flexion = curling in
- Extension = stretching
- Torsion toward anterior
- Torsion toward posterior

He elucidates in great detail the biomechanical processes in the individual areas of the spinal column, thorax, extremities, and cranium. **Chauffour draws an interesting connection between cranial biomechanics and parietal biomechanics.**

In another section of the book, Chauffour describes his diagnostic and therapeutic procedures. This involves very gentle fascial compression or traction tests.

Treatment consists of a kind of reflective impulse after the osteopath has performed a complete examination. For this impulse, the therapist detects the greatest resistance in the affected segment at all spatial planes and builds up a slight tension, to then execute the impulse. The most interesting part of this model are the myofascial explanations for the creation of dysfunctions.

In the following section, we do not present the individual chains, but limit ourselves to the explanations that Chauffour gives for the creation of dysfunctions in the individual segments, with reference to the cervical, thoracic, and lumbar vertebrae. Chauffour's myofascial chains are more or less identical to Leopold Busquet's.

Flexion Pattern

- C1: The dens axis prevents the flexion of C1.
- C2: This is under particular stress because C1 and the lower cervical spinal column (CSC) flex less.
- C7: This is no longer stabilized by ribs and experiences fascial pull by the central tendon.
- T4: This the lowest vertebra that experiences fascial pull by the central tendon. The pars horizontalis of the trapezius ends at T4, and the pars ascendens starts at T5.
- T6: The fascia thoracolumbalis has a solid attachment to T7 via the latissimus dorsi. As a consequence, T6 is stressed during flexion.
- T12: This is pulled caudally via the psoas.
- L1 and L2: The crura of the diaphragm exert a pull on L1 and L2.

Extension Pattern

- The region T1–T12 is compressed upward by the pull of the trapezius muscle and downward by the pull of the latissimus dorsi muscle.
- T7 is therefore particularly susceptible.

- T11 is also under particular pressure for the same reason.
- L2 is pulled by the diaphragm.

Torsion toward Anterior

- C6: For Chauffour, C7 acts like a thoracic vertebra but C6 like a cervical vertebra. The opposite rotation during torsion causes stress between C6 and C7.
- C7: C7 has no joint connection with the first rib and is therefore less stabilized.
- T4: The central tendon reaches to T4 and slows down the rotation of the upper thoracic spinal column (TSC) during torsion of the trunk.
- T6: The aponeurosis of the latissimus dorsi muscle is attached to T7. T6 is therefore more susceptible.
- T10: The tenth rib stabilizes T10, which is no longer the case for T11 and T12. Torsion is clearly noticeable between T10 and T11.

- T11: T12 is the center of torsion and therefore barely moves during torsion. Therefore, T11 is stressed.
- L2: The crura of the diaphragm pull L2 along into the torsion.

Torsion toward Posterior

- C1: This is stressed because the lateral inclination between C1 and C2 is opposite.
- C6: The same applies for C6 and C7.
- T6: The fascia thoracolumbalis exerts more pull on the lower spinal column up to and including T7. This can cause conflict between T6 and T7.
- T10: Since T11 turns further than T10, stress arises between T10 and T11.
- T12: The trapezius muscle is attached up to T12, and this vertebra is therefore pulled further into the torsion than L1.

2.6 Conclusion on the Different Models of Myofascial Chains

To our knowledge, Kabath was the first person to emphasize the significance of chains in the treatment of weak muscles. He explains this by the fact that the brain only knows motion processes, not individual muscles. Accordingly, Kabath defined a series of motion patterns, without describing continuous chains from head to foot. His treatment methods are based on neurophysiologic findings that have since become the foundation for other muscle energy techniques.

The first to speak of muscle chains that cover the entire body was Godelieve Struyff-Denys. For her, psychic factors are the key reason for the formation and development of dominating muscle chains. The outer form of the body is molded by internal influences. Function determines structure. The muscle chains described by Struyff-Denys find continuity in the cranium. The shape of the skull is influenced by the muscle chains. Because the dominance of muscle chains can be rooted in genetic causes, it is impossible to extinguish a dominant chain. The therapist can only achieve "balance within imbalance."

Thomas Myers presents probably the most complex system of muscle chains, in which it is difficult to detect motion patterns. In this context, we need to consider the fact that Rolfers emphasize different aspects than osteopaths.

The two French osteopaths Paul Chauffour and Leopold Busquet have presented interesting models. Paul Chauffour describes in great detail the biomechanics of the locomotor system and the cranium in different motion patterns. His holistic motion patterns that include cranial movements are interesting. Leopold Busquet deals more directly with the musculature in muscle chains. He also draws connections to the cranial system, without explaining the dysfunctions described by Sutherland explicitly with muscle chains. He elucidates visceral causes of parietal malposture by reference to fascial connections, that is, the suspension system of the organs. Depending on the particular dysfunction, the musculature is programmed in such a way that it forms an environment that is as ideal as possible for the function of the affected organ. Malpositions of the spinal column, as well as dysfunctions and pathologies of the joints and periarticular structures, are vividly explained by myofascial imbalances.

3 Physiology

In clinic, it is important that therapists are able to diagnose as precisely as possible the state of the tissue to be treated. Therefore, they must know the properties of the tissue components to treat with a specific aim.

3.1 Components of the Connective Tissue

Embryologically, the connective tissue develops from the mesoderm and forms wide-meshed cell connections with intercellular substance.

■ The Cells

These consist of local cells, connective tissue cells, and mobile cells:

Local Cells

- Fibroblasts and fibrocytes
- Reticular cells
- Lipocytes
- Chondroblasts and chondrocytes
- Osteoblasts and osteocytes

Mobile Cells

In contrast to local cells, which originate in the mesenchyme, mobile cells stem from bone marrow cells (hematopoietic stem cells):
- Macrophages
- Monocytes
- Histiocytes
- Mast cells
- Granulocytes
- Lymphocytes

Mobile cells play a key role in cellular defense mechanisms.

■ The Intercellular Substance

The intercellular substance, also called matrix, consists of all extracellular components of the connective tissue. In addition to water, it contains components that are produced by the connective tissue cells.

■ The Basic Substance

Mucopolysaccharides: the basic substance consists of proteoglycans and glucosaminoglycans, which connect collagen and elastic fibers and bind with water. They stabilize the connective tissue and give the tissue elasticity. They absorb some of the forces acting upon the tissue and ensure that the tissue assumes its original shape after strain. The connection of proteoglycans and glucosaminoglycans creates a stress field.

In the tissue, changes in pressure cause the cells to absorb or emit water. Thereby, tissue tension fluctuates, which is called **piezoelectric activity**. This piezoelectric activity stimulates the cells to synthesize and to orient the collagen molecules. This is a property that can be utilized by fascial treatment techniques.[111]

The Fibers

Fibers are divided into:
- Collagen fibers
- Elastic or reticular fibers
- Non-collagenous proteins

Collagen Fibers or Fibrils

Collagen, from the Greek word for glue, *kolla*, translates as "binding with glue." Collagen fibers give the tissue its white color. Besides water, they are the second largest component of the connective tissue. They consist of individual fibers twisted into spirals that can assume certain shapes depending on strain (pressure or pull). Collagen fibers are found in ligament, capsules, tendons, aponeuroses, muscle septs, cartilage, and intervertebral disks.

Functions
- Collagen gives the tissue stability.
- It absorbs tensile forces.
- It counteracts compressive forces.

Properties
- Collagen is characterized by great tensile strength.
- The molecules arrange themselves in the direction of the tensile or compressive forces to counteract these. If the tensile direction remains constant, the fibers align themselves parallel to each other (tendons, ligaments). If the tensile directions change, the fibers form a criss-cross pattern (aponeuroses).
- The thickness and stability of collagen fibers depends on the strain they are exposed to. Specific training or strain increase the thickness and resistance of collagen fibers.
- The turnover of collagen fibers takes about 300–500 days.

Elastic Fibers

These are found primarily in the loose connective tissue: in the skin, the vessels, in elastic cartilage, but also in tendons and ligaments. Elastic fibers contain the substance elastin, which is colored yellow. In vessels, the proportion of elastic fibers is 50%, in skin and tendons, roughly 5%. The ligamentum flavum consists primarily of elastic fibers and therefore has a yellow coloration.

Functions
- Elastic fibers give the tissue elasticity and mobility.
- In tendons and ligaments, they allow the collagen fibers to maintain their wave-shaped arrangement.
- Tensile and compressive forces are first absorbed by elastic fibers, to be then transferred evenly to collagen fibers.

Properties
- Elastic fibers consist of the shapeless substance elastin, surrounded by microfibrils. The elastic microfibrils are greatly ramified and contain frequent connections with each other. Thereby, they create a stretchable network. Elastic fibers can be stretched by more than 150%.
- The tear (tensile) strength of elastic fibers is around 300 Newtons per square centimeter (N/cm^2).
- The tensile strength of elastic fibers increases with stretching. The resistance increases incrementally.

Non-Collagenous Proteins

This refers to branching and connecting proteins that are found in the entire connective tissue. They can be produced by all connective tissue cells.

Functions
- They are in charge of connecting the extracellular components of the connective tissue to each other. In this way, a network is formed that allows the connective tissue to function properly.
- They participate in metabolic processes by facilitating the transport of substances through the connective tissue and influencing the polarity of cells.
- They form links between proteoglycans and hyaluronic acid chains, by which water can be bound in the tissue. The tissue can thereby fulfill its pressure-absorbing function.

Water

Approximately 60% of our body weight comes from water. Of this, 70% is intracellular and 30% extracellular. In the extracellular part, the water is distributed in the following areas:
- As interstitial fluid in the intercellular tissue
- As a component of blood in the vessels
- As a component of the liquor
- As axoplasmic fluid in the nerves

Functions
- Transport and solvent
- It gives tissue volume and shape.
- It has a shock absorber function.
- It plays a role in thermoregulation.
- It facilitates metabolic processes.

3.2 Supply of the Connective Tissue

The capillary vessels supply the tissue with nutrients and oxygen. Waste products are removed from the interstitium via veins and lymphatic vessels. In the tissue itself, the cells are supplied by diffusion and osmosis.

▪ Diffusion

This refers to the movement of substances to a location with a lower concentration. The amount of diffused matter depends on the concentration gradient, particle size, diffusion surface, tissue viscosity, and on the distance that the particles have to travel.

■ Osmosis

This is a type of diffusion in which a substance is moved through a semipermeable membrane to a location with higher concentration. The particles composing the substance with the higher concentration are too large to penetrate the pores in the membrane. The smaller particles diffuse to the large particles until concentration is balanced.

The vegetative nervous system plays an important role for permeability. Vegetative nervous cells release neurotransmitters that increase the permeability of the cell walls. In addition, neuropeptides stimulate the synthesis of adrenaline, noradrenaline, and acetyl-choline, as well as the release of pain substances, immunoglobulins, and histamine.

The formation and maintenance of connective tissue requires physiological strain.[12] Muscles, tendons, and ligaments need to be tensed and optimally stretched. Cartilages and disks need to be stimulated by compression and decompression.

Movement improves general blood circulation in the tissue and promotes piezoelectric activity. Both of these contribute to cell synthesis. For ligaments and tendons, it is important that they are stretched longitudinally, to stimulate the orientation of the collagen fibers.

3.3 The "Creep" Phenomenon

Creep is caused by the distortion of the collagenous network and fibrils. This presses fluid out of the tissue. Because this is a lengthy process, the duration of the pressure is a decisive factor. The pliability of the tissue is lost because the fluid content in the tissue is partly responsible for its malleability.

3.4 The Muscle

The smallest component of the muscle is the myofibril, which is divided into two parts: the actin and myosin filaments. These give the striated muscle its characteristic striped shape. Myofibrils are grouped in bundles of 100–200 and form skeletal muscle cells or muscle fibers. These range in average from 10–100 micrograms (μm).

The cell membrane of muscle fibers is called sarcolemma and encloses not only the myofibrils but also the sarcoplasm, several nuclei, mitochondria, lysosomes, glycogen granules, and fat droplets. The muscle fibers in turn are joined together into fiber bundles (100–1000 μm). They are surrounded by membranes that merge with the membranes of other fiber bundles into the tendons of the muscle. We distinguish between two types of muscles:
• Smooth musculature
• Striated musculature

The smooth musculature differs from the striated musculature in the following aspects:
1. It contains no cross-stripes. It consists of actin and myosin, but it lacks the thick filaments and sarcomeres.
2. Stimulation of the smooth musculature is autonomous:
   — First, by ion bridges (gap junctions), as is the case for most organs. The contraction of these muscles is predominantly independent of external nerve impulses. Stretching the muscle causes depolarization and thereby increases muscle tone = myogenic tone.
   — Alternatively, stimulation can come from vegetative nerves. Examples: iris, vas deferens, blood vessels (which, however, also have a myogenic tone).

3.5   The Fasciae

The fasciae are part of the connective tissue. Apart from the fasciae, a number of other tissues also belong to the connective tissue: subcutaneous tissue, skin, muscles, tendons, ligaments, and so on.

Connective tissue contains collagen, elastic, and reticular fibers, mucus cells, bone tissue, as well as cartilage cells. It is formed by fibroblasts, fibroglia, collagen fibers, and elastic fibers.

All body cells are surrounded by fasciae. Fasciae connect all cells to each other; they give the body support and shape.

■ Functions of the Fasciae

The fascial functions described below are generally referred to as "the Four Ps"[82]: packaging, protection, posture, and passageway.

Packaging

The fasciae form covers for all bodily structures. They separate individual structures from each other, but at the same time connect them. Their resistibility keeps them in place and characterizes their mobility.

Protection

By enclosing all organs, the fasciae provide support and protection to the structures. Varying degrees of tissue density give the structures their resistibility, keep them in place, and characterize their mobility.

Posture

Posture, that is, statics, is determined by the locomotor system. The proprioceptors are located in the body's fascial structures. Muscle spindles and Golgi tendon receptors in the muscles, as well as Pacini and Golgi corpuscles in the ligaments and capsules provide for postural tone and for necessary adjustments to postural changes induced from the outside. The muscles play an active role in this process, while the fasciae constitute a connecting element.

The fasciae contain great numbers of free nerve endings as well as pain receptors. Some authors (Becker,[8] Upledger[148]) attribute a memory function to the tissues. They surmise that certain motion patterns, traumas, and injuries are stored at the fascial level. It is still unclear how this happens. Biochemical, physical, and energetic processes are proposed as causative factors.

The connective tissue stores the energy of an injury in the form of "energy cysts." **This tissue change can be felt and treated by the therapist**.

Passageway

The fasciae form vessel passageways or pathways for nerves, arteries, veins, and lymphatic vessels. Secretory and excretory channels are made from connective tissue. For this reason, the fasciae play an important role in all metabolic processes. Because the connective tissue gives the organs their shape (liver, pituitary gland, adrenal gland) and forms vesicles that contain enzymes and hormones (gall bladder, lymph nodes), tensions in the fasciae can influence organ function and metabolism.

Homeostasis of the organism depends greatly on the condition of the connective tissue.

■ Manifestations of Fascial Disorders[40, 41, 82, 111, 113]

Somatic Disorders

Because of their influence on receptors, vessels, and nerves, fascial tensions initiate osteopathic lesions.

Metabolic Disorders

Tensions disturb circulation in the interstitium and thereby tissue metabolism. This leads to palpable changes in the tissue (trigger points, swellings, fibroses).

Fascial Disorders

These become evident in swellings. Certain regions are particularly susceptible: supraclavicular triangle, armpit, groin, back of the knee, epigastrium.

Changes in Breathing

Myofascial tensions affect posture as well as pressure conditions in the abdomen and thorax. This directly influences the function of the thoracic pump.

Postural Disorders

Posture is a compromise between stability and mobility in which the myofascial chains act like a generator. Wrong or excessive strain causes malpostures and malfunctions.

The Creation of Fascial Patterns

Certain fascial patterns are found in both healthy and sick people. The causes are unknown (congenital or acquired). In asymptomatic people, we find alternating fascial trains:

Occipitoatlantoaxial (OAA) complex	right → left
Cervicothoracic junction (CTJ)	left → right
Thoracolumbar junction (TLJ)	right → left
Lumbosacral junction (LSJ)	left → right

Zink found this pattern in 80% of all cases. In the remaining 20%, the fascial trains were present in the opposite direction.

In people with dysfunctions, we do not find this alternation. Instead, we find identical myofascial trains in two consecutive junctions.

Systemic Changes

Tissue tension affects the circulation of the tissue and therefore also the function of structures, resulting in functional and later structural damage.

▪ Evaluation of Fascial Tensions

Anamnesis provides clues regarding fascial tensions. The following also provide valuable clues:

- Observing posture: fascial tensions manifest in malposture (in the three planes of motion).
- Testing fascial preferences in the junctions: the place where the rotation is most noticeable indicates the dominant dysfunction.
- Palpating the tissue for contractures, fibroses, and swellings.
- Mobilizing the extremities to find muscular imbalances by comparison.

Note: The diaphragm is particularly important for myofascial chains because it is an active factor for the musculature as well as for circulation. In addition, it is the main regulator for pressure conditions in all body cavities.

▪ Causes of Musculoskeletal Dysfunctions

The following factors can cause myofascial changes (the order in which they are listed is not related to their significance):

- Postural imbalances
- Life habits, stress: work, relaxation
- Congenital malpositions: differences in leg length, scoliosis
- Perinatal trauma
- Emotional stress factors: intro-, extroverted
- Repetitive stretching, pulling during work or leisure activities
- Hypo-, hypermobile joints, rheumatic changes
- Traumas, inflammatory processes
- Infection
- Disease
- Immobilization
- Metabolic disorders, wrong diet (lack of Vitamin C affecting the formation of collagen fibers in the tissue)
- Nerve lesions due to changes in the trophic function of the nerves

▪ Genesis of Myofascial Disorders

Biochemical, biomechanical, and psychological dysfunctions can lead to stress situations for myofascial structures. Leon Chaitow[40] postulated that these changes could proceed as follows:

1. A functional disorder in the organism causes a local increase in muscle tone.
2. This increase in muscle tone leads to a reduced elimination of waste products and a local undersupply with oxygen, which in turn leads to ischemia (depending on strenuous activities of the muscle).
3. Increased tone can lead to local edemas.
4. These factors (waste products, ischemia, swelling) cause tension and pain.
5. Pain and tension cause or increase hypertonicity.
6. Inflammation, or at least chronic irritation, can result.
7. This causes a segmental facilitation at the level of the spinal cord.
8. Macrophages and fibroblasts are activated.
9. Production of connective tissue increases, with the formation of so-called "links," which causes induration and shortening.

10. Because of the continuity of the fasciae, tension arises in other areas of the organism, affecting lymph and blood circulation.
11. Fibrosis of the muscle tissue occurs as a result of vascular disturbances.
12. In a chain reaction, this makes the postural muscles shorter and the phasic muscles weaker.
13. Shortened muscles lead to tensions of the tendons with pain in the periosteum.
14. Muscular imbalances affect movement coordination.
15. This results in articular dysfunctions as well as further fascial changes.
16. Segmental facilitation on the spinal cord level progresses further and further, and trigger points are formed in the muscles.
17. Muscle contractures cause a loss of energy.
18. Other bodily systems are burdened by the hypertonicity, for example, respiratory function and digestion.
19. In the long run, hypertonicity, muscle shortening, and neural facilitation cause increased sympathetic tone and negative feedback in the central nervous system (CNS). This results in internal unrest and irritability, which in turn further increases tension.
20. In this state, other functional disturbances can occur.
21. This opens the door for acute pathologies. The person is no longer able to help themselves out of their misery.

The pains associated with this process are explained by the release of tissue hormones. Bradykinin, histamine, serotonin, and prostaglandin stimulate alpha, delta, and C fibers. Furthermore, the limbic system and the frontal lobes of the cerebrum are involved.

The perception of pain varies from one person to the next and also differs depending on the situation. Studies[2, 40, 41, 79, 113] were able to demonstrate that emotional stress lowers the pain threshold in the same way as infections.

When stimuli like microtraumas affect the organism progressively, the pain threshold is more likely to be raised. Acute traumas, on the other hand, lower it. This is related to the fact that the body attempts to keep nociceptive stimulation ineffective for as long as possible because of their damaging effect (release of tissue hormones, inflammation, release of macrophages, fibroses, and so on). We should also mention in this context that pain pathways are quick conductors, while the pathways that conduct impulses from the joints are slow.

■ Patterns of Pain

If a person indicates pain in a certain area of the body, this can be a manifestation of a number of phenomena: radicular pain, referred pain syndrome, pseudoradicular pain, myofascialtrigger points, tender points, or viscerosomatic reflexes.

Radicular Pain

* The pain area corresponds to the regions supplied by the segment.
* There is disturbed sensitivity in the supplied areas.
* Sometimes loss of strength occurs in the muscles supplied by the segment, to the point of atrophy.
* Weakening of tendon reflexes occurs.

Referred Pain Syndrome

Expression for pain that is not radicular, but projected, for example, Head's areas.

Pseudoradicular Pain

Pain radiating out into certain skin regions, caused by irritation of a peripheral nerve, for example femoral neuralgia due to psoas muscle contracture.

Tender Points

This refers to pressure-sensitive points (indurations) at certain areas of the locomotor system. The origination of such points is related to pulled or stretched muscles or stress on the motor system.[40, 43, 82, 145, 156] These points are not always located in the areas indicated as painful by the patient. The points serve as diagnostic tool and as indicators for treatment efficacy.

Viscerosomatic Reflexes[35, 46, 79, 82, 156]

Somatic dysfunctions in the organs send afferent impulses to the posterior horn of the spinal column, where they communicate with interneurons. These stimuli are then transmitted by motor and sympathetic fibers to the muscles, skin, and vessels.

These abnormal stimuli can result in hypersensitivity of the skin, vasoconstriction, or increased sudomotor activity. Simultaneously, muscular hypertonicity can arise in the muscles supplied motorically by the segment.

This viscerosomatic reflex activity generally already exists before the organ in question manifests any symptoms. Changes in the skin or in sweat production, as well as hypertonicity of the paravertebral musculature are diagnostically of great value. When this pathology becomes chronic, structural changes in the tissue occur: the skin becomes "furry" and the muscles tend towards fibrosis. The distinctness of these symptoms is directly related to the intensity of organ pathology.

As a rule, several segments are limited in their mobility when the cause is a viscerosomatic reflex.

Trigger Points[38, 40, 43, 82, 145, 156]

A trigger point is a palpable mass in the muscle tissue that is tender on pressure. The pain is local and radiates out into a predictable region, in the same way in every person. Trigger points are similar to spinal column segments in that they are "facilitated" areas of the musculature, that is, they can be activated by often-subliminal stimuli.

In general, trigger points are located in tightened fibers of the affected muscle, mostly near the base of the muscle. Affected muscle fibers can be snapped with the finger, like strings on a guitar.

Note: Some types of hysteria with impaired vision, respiratory disturbances, or motoric breakdown, as well as insensitivity, can stem from impulses that originate in trigger points. It is a fact that hysterical people tend to have trigger points.

As another possible result, active trigger points can cause the formation of silent or latent trigger points in the muscles of the region into which the active trigger points radiates. This could possibly explain the snowball effect in certain pain syndromes.

Notes:
- According to Melzack and Wall, ± 80% of all acupuncture points are active and inactive trigger points.[38, 40]
- Lawrence Jones' tender points are for many authors no more than inactive trigger points.[40, 145]
- Emotional factors are the strongest stimuli for the formation and activation of trigger points.
- Certain muscles (e.g., trapezius, pectoralis, piriformis) are more frequently affected by trigger points.
- Treatment varies and includes:
  - injections
  - acupuncture needles
  - cooling spray
  - friction, acupressure
  - myofascial release
  - muscle energy technique (MET)
  - strain/counterstrain method
  - positional release technique

We will elaborate on some of these treatment techniques below.

3.6   Vegetative Innervation of the Organs

In this section, we present a brief overview of the segmental supply of the organs. Via viscerosomatic reflexes, organ dysfunctions can be starting points for postural imbalances and restricted mobility:

Eyes:	T1–T4
Lacrimal and salivary glands:	T1–T4
Paranasal sinuses:	T1–T4
Carotid sinus and glomus:	T1–T4
Thyroid:	T1–T4
Trachea:	T1–T6
Bronchial tubes:	T1–T6
Esophagus:	T1–T6
Cardia:	T5–T6
Mammary glands:	T1–T6
Aorta:	T1–T6
Heart:	T1–T6
Lungs:	T1–T6
Stomach:	T6–T9
Pylorus:	T9
Liver:	T5–T9
Gallbladder and bile ducts:	T6–T9
Spleen:	T6–T9
Pancreas:	T6–T10

Duodenum, upper part:	T6–T9
Duodenum, lower part:	T10–T11
Small intestine:	T9–T11
Large intestine total:	T10–L2
Cecum:	T11–T12
Ascending colon:	T11–L1
Descending colon:	L1–L2
Adrenal gland:	T10–T11
Kidneys:	T10–T11
Ureter:	T11–L1
Bladder:	T12–L2
Prostate:	T12–L2
Sigmoid colon:	L1–L2
Rectum:	L1–L2
Uterus:	T12–L2
Ovaries:	T10–T11
Testicles:	T10–T11
Upper extremity:	T2–T8
Lower extremity:	T9–L2

3.7   Irvin M. Korr

If there is one non-osteopath who deserves the gratitude and recognition of osteopaths, this is surely Irvin M. Korr. In addition to Louisa Burns and John Stedman Denslow, Korr contributed in over 50 years of research to the collection of scientific evidence for the causes and results of osteopathic lesions. It is largely to his credit that a vertebral blockage is no longer seen only as a blockage of the joint, but as a neuromusculoarticular dysfunction.

In the framework of this book, it is impossible to give even an overview of Korr's work. We therefore limit ourselves to those research findings that appear important for the subject of this book. For the interested reader, we can only recommend *The Collected Papers of Irvin M. Korr, Vols I–II.*[79]

■ Significance of a Somatic Dysfunction in the Spinal Column for the Entire Organism

A somatic dysfunction in the spinal column:
- Leads to hypertonicity of the paravertebral musculature around the affected segment
- Results in an elevated sympathetic tone of the segment
- Affects the conductivity of the nerves
- Lowers the stimulus threshold of all receptors that depend on this segment

Korr coined the terms "facilitated segment" and "neurologic lens."

Facilitated Segment

A somatic dysfunction in the spinal column causes a lowered stimulus threshold of all centers of the affected segment.

Neurologic Lens

Because of the low stimulus threshold of the receptors, the facilitated segment becomes susceptible to weaker stimuli. This has two types of effects:

- Cerebral impulses (emotions, stress, fear, anger) reach the stimulus threshold of these segments more easily and therefore trigger symptoms here more quickly (see stomach aches in stress).
- Stimuli that under normal circumstances only reach neighboring segments can also affect the facilitated segment.

■ Significance of the Spinal Cord

The Spinal Cord as Information and Control Center

Spinal cord segments receive information from the brain as well as from the periphery. Likewise, pathways go from the spinal cord to the brain and to the peripheral structures. On the level of the spinal cord, all centers are connected to each other via interneurons. All inputs stimulate or inhibit each other, giving an output adjusted to the momentary needs.

The spinal cord is that part of the central nervous system that receives the most afferences. The afferences that arrive in a segment of the spinal cord are also connected to neighboring segments via interneurons. This is important, for example, for the execution of harmonious movements. In this way, agonists, synergists, and stabilizers can be activated at the same time that their antagonists are inhibited.

The Spinal Cord as Reflex Center

A multitude of vital reflexes are spinal reflexes (flexion reflex, crossed extensor reflex, tendon reflex, and so on). They are part of plastic motion patterns of daily life (running, dancing, swimming). This minimizes strain on the brain.

The Spinal Cord Segment as Starting Point for Functions

In order to carry out a movement, relevant muscles must be activated and also vascularized sufficiently and so on. This is coordinated at the multi-segmental level.

■ Significance of the Autonomous Nervous System

On the basis of a series of experiments, Korr was able to demonstrate the negative influence of continuing high sympathetic tone on human health:

- The sympathetic nervous system increases muscle strength and reduces muscle fatigue.
- Receptor sensitivity is increased, the stimulus threshold is lowered.
- The sympathetic nervous system influences neural irritability and brain activity.
- The sympathetic nervous system modulates the metabolism. Bone growth, lipolysis, and erythropoiesis *are stimulated.*
- The entire endocrine system is under the influence of the sympathetic nervous system.

These are all vital processes that nevertheless have detrimental effects in the case of continuing high sympathetic tone.

■ Significance of the Nerves for Trophism

In addition to nerve impulses, the nerves also serve as pathways for peptides, which are necessary for tissue growth. Korr was able to demonstrate experimentally how denervation can lead to atrophy.

In other experiments, Korr's team was able to illustrate how quickly postural imbalances stimulate the sympathetic nervous system in certain areas of the spinal column. The first vegetative manifestations were noticeable as early as 1 hour after the occurrence of an imbalance.

Also noteworthy is the recognition of the extreme sensitivity of muscle spindles. A muscle spindle reacts to a pull of 1 g and a stretch of 1/1000 mm. This makes the muscle spindle one of the most sensitive organs in the human body.

Other researchers have also investigated the topic of "somatic dysfunction":

- J.S. Denslow[2] was able to demonstrate that the paravertebral muscles in blocked segments are more irritable and therefore react to lower stimuli. These muscles react to a stimulus with a stronger contraction.
- Louisa Burns[2] studied the effects of somatic dysfunctions on muscles and organs. She found microscopic tissue changes already after 96 hours.
- Michael Patterson[112] explained that continuous facilitation leads to chronic lesions.
- Akio Sato[82, 112] was able to show experimentally somatovisceral reflex pathways. Somatic dysfunctions cause organic malfunctions.

In conclusion, we can say that these researchers were able to prove that somatic dysfunctions in the spinal column cause a lowered stimulus threshold in the segments and that this stimulates the sympathetic nervous system, which in turn causes visceral malfunctions. If this facilitated state persists for a longer period of time, it can make the problem chronic. Due to the sensitivity of the muscle spindles, the muscles play a key role in this process.

The significance of the nervous system as switching and coordination center is made clear. The CNS coordinates all functions of the entire organism, as well as all adaptations in the case of dysfunctions. Therefore, the spinal column plays a central role for both diagnosis and for treatment.

3.8 Sir Charles Sherrington

Sir Charles Sherrington was a neurophysiologist who at the beginning of the 20th century (1906) published a number of interesting research findings (*The Integrative Action of the Nervous System*, Yale University Press, New Haven). His discoveries have not only contributed to our understanding of the formation of motion patterns; we also have to thank him for **neurophysiological explanations** for the effectiveness of certain muscle techniques.

■ Inhibition of the Antagonist or Reciprocal Innervation (or Inhibition)

Stimulation of the agonist leads to simultaneous inhibition of the antagonist and activation of the synergist.

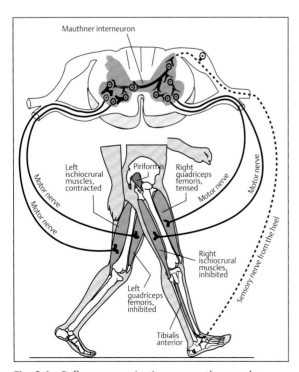

Fig. 3.1 Reflex communication among the muscles.

■ Post-isometric Relaxation

After being tensed, muscle fibers can more easily be relaxed and stretched. This relaxation stage can last up to 15 seconds.

■ Temporary Summation and Local, Spatial Summation

Temporary or local summation of several supra- or subliminal single stimuli causes an impulse or effect that cannot be evoked by single stimulus.

■ Successive Induction

The irritability of antagonists is increased immediately after contraction of the agonist.

These are only a few of the physiological facts described by Sherrington that must be taken into consideration in the application of muscle techniques.

A further physiological principle plays a key role in posture and motion patterns: **the crossed stretch reflex**. This refers to a defense or flight reflex. Irritation of the sole of the right foot by a pain impulse for example, leads to flexion of the hip, knee, and foot. At the same time, the extensors of the left leg are stimulated via interneurons.

We find the same phenomenon in certain motion patterns, such as the gait (**Fig. 3.1**). F.L. Mitchell Jr. describes a similar phenomenon in cases of somatic dysfunction.[107]

Example: In the case of a right anterior ilium, the muscles that turn the ilium forward dominate on the right side. The crossed stretch reflex causes an activation of those muscles on the left side that turn the ilium dorsally. This makes the malpositions even more obvious.

3.9   Harrison H. Fryette[56, 121, 125]

Harrison H. Fryette, one of Still's most brilliant students, is known among all osteopaths for his analysis of spinal biomechanics. Since their publication in the 1920s, "Fryette's Laws" have been the fundamental explanatory model for the physiology of the spinal column. In spite of the fact that the validity of Fryette's Laws have been questioned by numerous expert manual therapists, we do have to give him credit for providing an explanatory model for the formation of osteopathic lesions that functions in clinic. His achievement is even more noteworthy when we consider that he did not have access to any imaging techniques for his studies.

Osteopathic dysfunctions are very complex processes shaped also by causes other than mechanical factors. We are dealing with living tissue with specific properties (plasticity, hydrolytic properties, piezoelectricity). This and the fact that all movement is three-dimensional, wherein movement amplitudes can differ in the individual levels, make any regulatory statement risky. In spite of all this, Fryette's model is a useful model in clinic, at least from a purely mechanical perspective.

Examining our patients, we find segmental dysfunctions and group lesions as described by Dr. Fryette. In motion tests, we can palpate the behavior of the vertebrae and recognize Fryette's Laws. It appeared normal to us that this was often impossible, because congenital or acquired anomalies as well as traumas are common.

▪ Lovett's Laws

In 1907, another physician, Robert A. Lovett, published a text in which he described the physiology of the spinal column. For his studies, Lovett separated the vertebral arches from the vertebral bodies, analyzed the behavior of each column under strain (lumbar [LSC], thoracic [TSC] and cervical [CSC]), and deducted the following rules:
- LSC: If the LSC is forced into a sideways bend, the vertebrae rotate into the concavity.
- TSC: When the TSC makes a sideways bend, the thoracic vertebrae always turn into the convexity.
- CSC: Sidebending causes rotation into the concavity.

Because this was not always confirmed in practice, Fryette investigated the mechanics of the spinal column from a different angle. He thereby realized that the behavior of the vertebrae differed, depending on whether the facets of the zygapophyseal joints were in contact or not. He found out that all vertebrae below C2 correspond in sidebending and rotation, if the joint facets are in contact. When no contact exists, the vertebrae have opposite rotation and sidebending.

The starting point for a movement is essential for determining whether or not the joint surfaces of the arch joints touch each other. Other factors are the curvature of the spinal column and the orientation of the joint surfaces.

Lumbar Spinal Column

- The LSC is concave posteriorly.
- The facets stand almost vertical in the sagittal plane. Isolated rotation and sidebending are therefore limited, and facet contact occurs very early. Flexion of the LSC leads to early contact of the joint surfaces. During extension, on the other hand, contact occurs relatively late.

Thoracic Spinal Column

- The TSC is convex posteriorly.
- The facets are oriented outward posteriorly and lie almost in a frontal plane. Due to the position of the facets and the kyphosis of the CSC, extension is the earliest parameter that leads to facet contact.

Cervical Spinal Column

- The CSC is lordotic.
- The facets are oriented outward posteriorly and are influenced in their position by the lordosis. In the lower CSC (C5–C7), their vertical position is very pronounced; in the central and upper CSC clearly less so.
- The uncinate processes and saddle shape of the cervical plateau, however, only allow for matching rotation and sidebending of the cervical vertebrae.
- The OAA complex has its own physiology (atypical vertebra).

■ Fryette's Laws

First Law: Neutral Position–Sidebending–Rotation

Fryette called the neutral position "easy-flexion." This refers to the range of motion in the sagittal plane between the points where facet contact occurs in flexion and extension.

When the spinal column makes a sideways bend from the neutral position, the vertebrae rotate into the newly formed convexity (**Fig. 3.2**). This affects several vertebrae.

Second Law: Flexion(or Extension)–Rotation–Sidebending

When the spinal column makes a sideways bend from a flexion or extension position in which the facets are in contact, the vertebrae are forced to make a rotation to the same side (**Fig. 3.3**). This is due to the orientation of the joint plane. This movement can be executed by a group of vertebrae, but also in isolation.

These are physiological movements of the spinal column that we execute on a daily basis:

• In every step, the LSC and TSC make neutral position–sidebending–rotation (NSR) movements and the CSC makes extension–rotation–sidebending (ERS) movements.

• Every time we bend sideways out of a stoop, at least one vertebra makes a flexion–rotation–sidebending (FRS) movement.

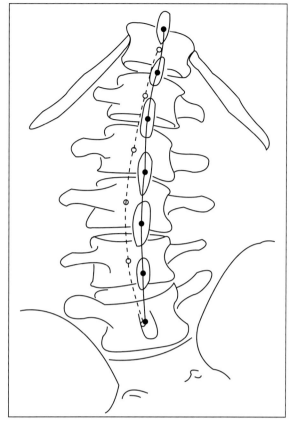

Fig. 3.2 Behavior of the lumbar vertebrae during sidebending from the neutral position (NSR). Adaptive lumbar curvature.

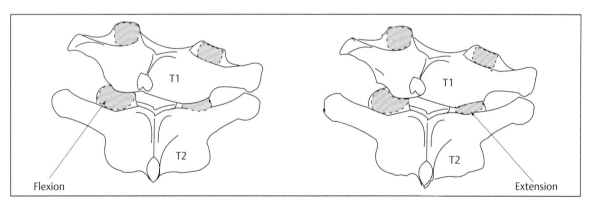

Fig. 3.3 Facet position in flexion and extension.

3.10　The Gait as a Global Functional Motion Pattern

The gait is perhaps the most impressive example for an activity that affects the entire body. We can see here how the entire locomotor system acts according to a certain pattern (motion pattern).[10, 19, 63, 107] All myofascial structures and all joints act as propelling organ as well as shock absorber.

The physiological processes of twisting together and twisting apart that occurs in the legs and trunk follow a special pattern. With the forward impulse during walking, this leads to the conversion of chemical energy, created by muscle activity, to kinetic energy that propels the body forward.[155] We can compare this motion pattern to a spring that unwinds when the leg swings and winds back up when the weight once again lands on the heel. The impulse in the gait starts when the heel touches the floor, the weight is shifted forward, and the leg muscles conduct the movement through the pelvis towards the spinal column.

The fact that almost all joints permit three-dimensional movement, together with the alternating order of lordoses and kyphoses from the sole of the foot up to the root of the nose, and the arrangement of muscles into *lemnisci* permit harmonious and economical locomotion. **This illustrates how function depends on structure**.

Note: In an interesting article, Gracovetsky (in [155]) sets forth the hypothesis that the anteroposterior curves of the spinal column are not only an adaptation to gravity, but also serve the function of making locomotion more economical. Kypholordoses act like an anteroposterior leaf spring that is pressed together when the foot is set down and stretches out when the leg swings.

Howard J. Dananberg, posturologist and director of the Walking Clinic in New Hampshire, United States, describes impressively in an article titled "Lower Back Pain as a Gait-related Repetitive Motion Injury" (in [155]) how an extension deficit in the metatarsophalangeal (MTP) joint of the large toe can be the starting point for lumbar pain.

A stretch deficit of the large toe prevents the foot from rolling off completely during walking. The organism compensates for this by increasing the dorsal extension of the foot, flexing the knee, and flexing the hip. The result is an imbalance between hip benders and hip stretchers, which shortens the length of the stride. The iliopsoas and quadratus lumborum muscles in turn balance this out with an increased pelvis rotation. This example shows how a foot lesion is compensated with a certain muscle chain, which can lead to a predictable dysfunction.

▪ Gait Analysis

Here, we reproduce a description of the gait cycle as most experts view it. The gait cycle (**Fig. 3.4a–f**) can be divided into several stages. We limit our account to describing two stages:

- Swing stage
- Stance stage

Both stages occur simultaneously, with one leg being the stance leg and the other the swing leg. The body weight is balanced on the stance leg, as a result of which the other leg can be propelled forward (**Fig. 3.5a–c**).

Due to the forward swinging of one leg, the pelvis is rotated to the stance leg. This leads to a counter-rotation to the side of the swing leg at the TLJ. We can recognize this from the arm movements, which are opposite to the leg movements.

During the swing stage, the hip is bent and the foot extended dorsally, while the knee is bent in the first half and stretched in the second half, before the heel touches the ground.

In the stance stage (**Fig. 3.5d–f**), the hip is stretched. The knee is initially slightly bent, before being stretched completely. The stance stage begins at that moment when the heel first touches the ground. Afterwards, the foot is rolled off from the heel up to the large toe (**Fig. 3.5g–i**).

At this point, the lower ankle joint takes on a special role. A dysfunction here will change the entire gait cycle. The opposing movements at the pelvic girdle and the shoulder girdle result in minimal movement of the head and the ability to keep the vision straight ahead.

During walking, the spinal column makes a snaking or "scoliotic" movement, as a result of which the LSC is brought convex to the swing side, while the TSC is brought convex to the stance side.

The pelvis makes a global rotation toward the stance side and a slight tilt to the swing side. During the gait cycle, changes also occur in the pelvis itself between the sacrum and ilium. In this context, the pubic symphysis plays the role of a half-mobile rotational pivot. In the symphysis itself, rotations take place in accordance with the iliac rotations.

Let us use the swing stage of the right leg as an example. This cycle begins in the moment when the left heel touches the ground and the right large toe loses contact with the ground. This orients the left ilium dorsally and the right one ventrally. The sacrum is in the neutral position between the two iliums. As soon as the right foot leaves the ground, weight is placed on the left leg. This causes a ligamentous (and

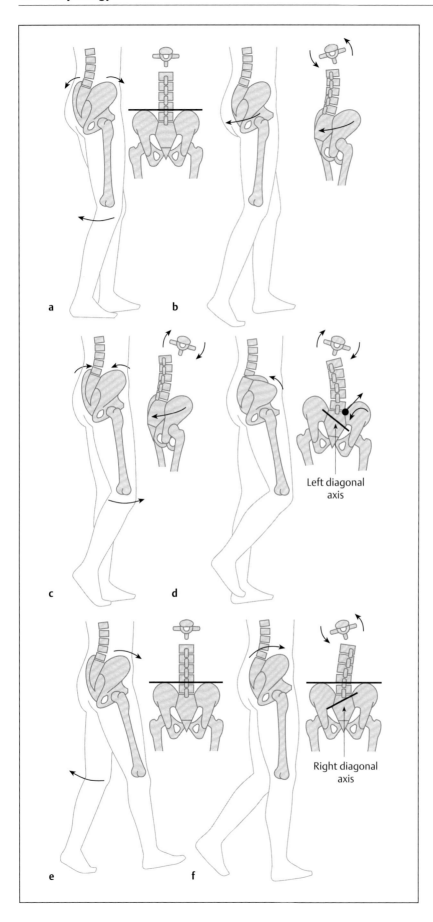

Fig. 3.4a–f Biomechanics and pelvic movements during each stage of the gait cycle.

a

b

c

d

Left diagonal
axis

e

f

Right diagonal
axis

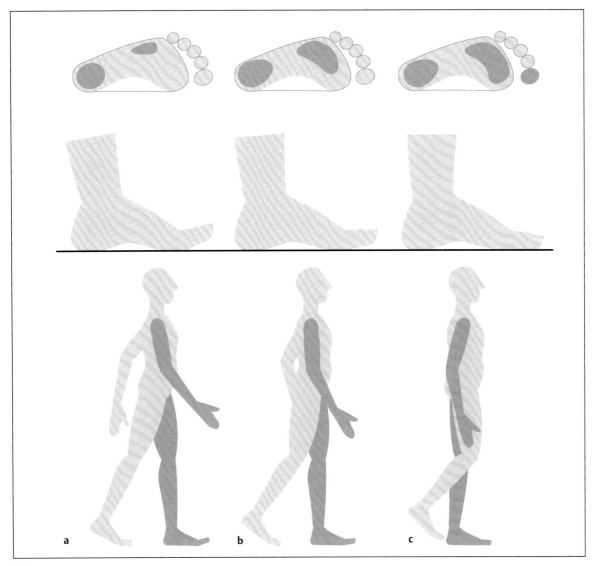

Fig. 3.5a–c Weight shifts during the stages of the gait cycle.

muscular) locking of the left iliosacral joint (ISJ) that contributes to stabilizing the body.

To shift the weight to the left leg, the LSC makes a leftward sidebend, which shifts pressure to the short shank of the left ISJ. Concurrently, the pelvis tips to the right (according to Schiowitz[49] by 5°). The lower pole of the right ISJ is compromised by the weight of the right leg and the resulting muscle tension. This causes a left diagonal axis. The LSC is in a neutral position with a leftward sidebend and rightward rotation (NSR according to Fryette). The sacrum below it makes a leftward rotation around a left diagonal axis (according to Mitchell[107]). The iliums rotate together with the spinal column, which guarantees constant tension in the ligaments.

During the swing stage of the right and the propelling stage of the left leg, the iliums rotate in the opposite direction. The right ilium rotates backward, the left one forward. This movement is initiated by muscles and completed by the momentum of the movement (the law of economy is observed).

Note: The sacrum moves in conjunction with the iliums, makes the same rotation and sidebend, but more slowly. As a result, it acquires the function of a ball-bearing that maintains the force lines between the spinal column and the two iliums.

■ Muscle Activity during Walking

For obvious reasons, we cannot describe muscle activity in detail here. First, statements in the literature regarding the activity of individual muscles vary widely. Second, muscle chains are, in our opinion, more important than isolated muscles. Furthermore, analysis is difficult because some joints have to be stabilized

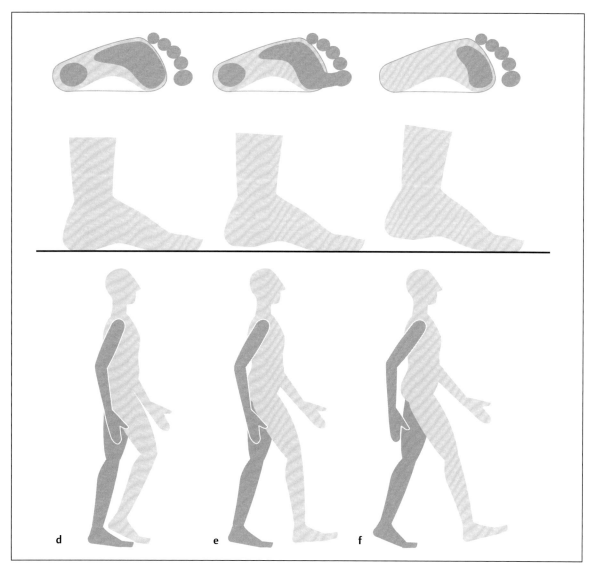

Fig. 3.5d–f Weight shifts during the stages of the gait cycle.

in several planes and movements take place three-dimensionally. Nevertheless, we describe the functions of individual muscles in the second half of this book on trigger points.

A classic example for muscle activity is the knee joint at the beginning of the stance stage. The ischii muscles and the quadriceps muscle stabilize the knee in the sagittal plane. The muscles of the pes anserinus prevent valgus of the knee. The iliotibial tract is tensed because the tensor fasciae latae (TFL) assists in preventing adduction of the hip.

Swing Stage

At the onset of the swing stage, when the large toe leaves the ground, the iliopsoas and rectus femoris muscles bend the hip, while the ischiocrural muscle group bends the knee. The tibialis anterior lifts the foot together with the toe extensors. At the conclusion of the swing stage, the quadriceps extends the knee. Shortly before and during the moment when the heel touches the ground, the knee stabilizers are activated (see above). The swing leg stage therefore consists of an activation of the leg flexors.

Stance Stage

This stage begins when the heel touches the ground. The hip is flexed, the knee is stretched, and the foot and toes are extended dorsally. The stance leg has two functions to fulfill:
• Maintaining the stability of leg and pelvis (abductors)
• Propelling the upper body forward (extensors)

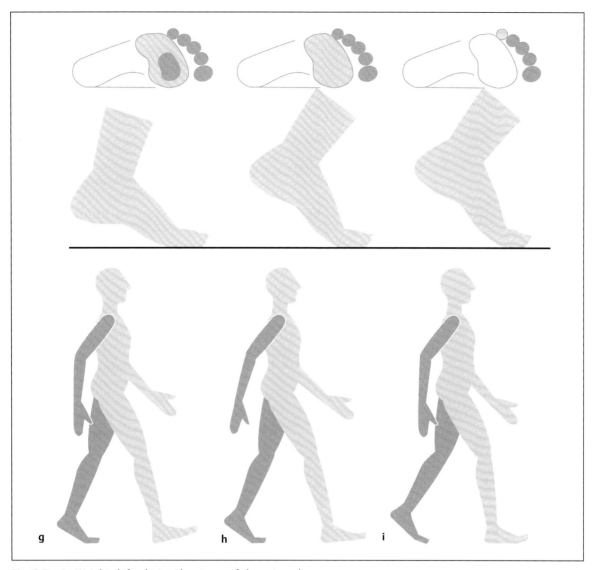

Fig. 3.5g–i Weight shifts during the stages of the gait cycle.

The stability of the pelvis is guaranteed by the gluteal muscles, the TFL, and the iliotibial tract. The valgus of the knee is guaranteed by the pes anserine muscles and by the chain of the muscles gluteus maximus–vastus lateralis–patellar retinaculum. The varus of the foot is limited by the peroneal muscles. This chain is continued towards the head via the gluteal muscles to the latissimus dorsi of the opposite side.

The upper body is propelled forward by a stretch in the hip, knee, and foot. The main muscles responsible for this action are the gluteus maximus quadriceps, triceps surae, and tibialis posterior, the peronei muscles, and the toe flexors.

An interesting insight is the fact that the muscles that are activated in one movement stage are positioned optimally by the preceding stage, that is, they are brought into a stretched position. The opposite rotation of pelvis and shoulder girdles as well as the opposite movement of the arms and legs illustrate this clearly.

When the right iliopsoas is supposed to pull the right hip forward, the left latissimus dorsi pulls the left arm backward and thereby stabilizes the spinal column, which gives the psoas a stable basis.

Ceccaldi and Favre[36] present the gait as a harmonious interplay of muscle chains in their book *Les Pivots Ostéopathiques*. The entire locomotor system behaves according to the same pattern that repeats itself with every pace. The pelvis and spinal column make certain movements around the pivots that had been described by J.M. Littlejohn. These two authors extend Littlejohn's model to the extremities and describe additional pivot points in the sternocostoclavicular joint, in the knee joint, and in the lower ankle joint.

As already mentioned above, the spinal column makes a scoliotic movement when the pelvis bends sideways during the swing stage. In this process, the lumbar vertebrae rotate to the side of the swing leg and the thoracic vertebrae to the side of the stance leg, with L3 and T6 being the respective apex of the turns. The CSC makes a translation to the swing leg side while rotating to the other side (Fryette II; see Fryette's Laws, p. 38 [in[107]]). This behavior can be illustrated with the hip drop test. This test imitates the gait cycle. We describe the behavior of the extremities in the section on muscle chains (see pp. 78ff)

By recalling W.G. Sutherland's craniosacral model, we can deduce the movements that the sphenobasilar synchondrosis (SBS) and the entire head make during every stride.

▪ Conclusion

The gait is a physiological function of the entire locomotor system in which the organism acts like a spring. The opposite arrangement of lordoses and kyphosis from the sole of the foot to the head, and the elasticity of the ligaments, tendons, and fasciae make it possible to release the energy won during the stance stage for the swing stage. This ensures that the law of economy is observed.

The gait cycle illustrates the two motion patterns. Flexion and extension alternate rhythmically. While the extensor chain is active on one side, the flexor chain dominates on the other side (Sherrington II; see the law of reciprocal innervation, p. 36 [in[107]]). This causes a torsion pattern of the spinal column (opposite rotation of the pelvic and shoulder girdles). From a craniosacral perspective, this results in torsions of the SBS.

Normally functioning structures are the precondition for a harmonious movement process. Hypo-, as well as hypermobility affect the motion pattern. The result is wrong postural as well as motoric behaviors.

Example: A dysfunction of the first metatarsal bone towards dorsal or of the talus towards anterior prevents the foot from rolling off, which over time causes a bent position of the lower extremity. The resulting shortening of the psoas cannot but affect the entire spinal column.

The motion pattern that the therapist finds in a patient corresponds to the adaptive pattern of the entire organism to its dysfunction. This phenomenon accords with the law of economy and painlessness, as well as the law of globality.

Note:

• Vleeming et al.[155] assume that the reason for premature exhaustion during slow walking, as for example during window shopping, is found in the fact that the spring principle cannot be applied here. As a result, the muscles, in particular those that are already overburdened by malposture and imbalance, have to work harder.

• H.J. Dananberg makes some interesting statements about the gait cycle in his article (in [155]). Walking is a daily activity. Considering that a person walks for an average of 80 minutes every day, which translates into around 2500 strides, this makes a total of around 1 000 000 strides per year. Certain occupations or sports can double or even triple this number. Even minor imbalances can cause pain symptoms.

• In another article (in [155]), Gracovetsky posits that the reason for the special biomechanics of the CSC could be that it neutralizes the rotation of the shoulder girdle in order to maintain a forward vision.

4   The Craniosacral Model

4.1   William G. Sutherland[54, 89, 101, 102, 136, 142, 143, 144]

There is no longer any need to introduce osteopaths to William G. Sutherland. All therapists who apply cranial osteopathy in their treatments will most likely have heard of him. Hence, we do not want to present Sutherland's life and work here, but merely those aspects that fit within the framework of this book.

Among Still's students, William G. Sutherland was probably the one who came closest to the master in his work. On the one hand, he recognized the significance of anatomy and biomechanics in the formation and treatment of dysfunctions. On the other hand, however, he was also aware that other factors exist that influence a person's health. Just like Still, Sutherland was a religious man who allowed this to influence his treatments. The "breath of life," as he called it, flows through the entire body via the liquor and interstitial fluid. This was an important aspect of Sutherland's treatment method.

In the course of his osteopathic work, Sutherland went through a remarkable development. Originally, the mechanical aspect clearly dominated in his treatments. We can see this from the fact that he considered cranial lesions as mechanical malpositions and treated them accordingly in his student years. As a result, he developed a kind of turban or helmet to influence individual cranial regions specifically. He also compared the bones of the cranial base with the vertebrae, and the cranial roof with the transverse and spinous processes.

In the same way that we can deduce the position of vertebral bodies from the position of the spinous and transverse processes, the cranial roof can inform us about the position of the sphenoid and occiput.

Embryologically, we can consider the cranium to consist of three modified vertebrae, with the occiput, sphenoid, and presphenoid (ethmoid) extending the

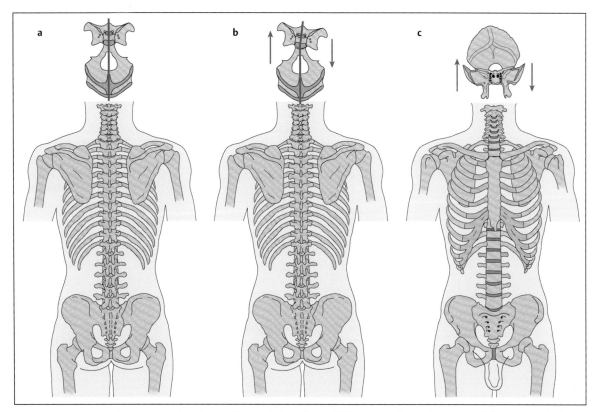

Fig. 4.1a–c   a Cranial "vertebra," **b** rightward bend of the sphenoidal bone, **c** rightward rotation of the sphenoidal bone.

spinal column towards the cranium. The occiput and sphenoid thereby form a frontally concave curve that is comparable with the thoracic spinal column (TSC) kyphosis.

In his terminology of movements, Sutherland used the same terms for the spinal column and the cranium (flexion, extension, torsion, and sidebending rotation), with sidebending rotation corresponding to extension–rotation–sidebending (ERS) or flexion–rotation–sidebending (FRS) (see Chapter 3).

The embryonic development of the brain and head is responsible for the fact that the planes of movement in rotation and sidebending differ for the sphenobasilar synchondrosis (SBS). In the course of philogenesis, the head bent forward to direct vision forward in the upright position.

While the rotation of the sphenoidal and occipital bones takes place in a frontal plane, they bend around a vertical axis into a transversal plane in sidebending rotation. Flexion and extension take place in a sagittal plane (**Fig. 4.1**).

Long years of practical experience and experiments caused Dr. Sutherland over time to change his treatment methods and treat more and more gently. Hence, he realized that dysfunctions can also be treated indirectly by bringing the affected joint or bone into a position that is as relaxed as possible and then letting the body do the correcting.

At the end of his career, Sutherland used the liquor—or the tides—for therapeutic purposes, by directing the liquor flow and utilizing respiration and movements of the extremities for support.

4.2   Biomechanics of the Craniosacral System

The theory of the craniosacral mechanism is based on five elements:
1. The motility of the nervous system
2. The fluctuation of the cerebrospinal fluid (CSF)
3. The reciprocal tension membranes: falx, tentorium (**Fig. 4.2**), and dura mater
4. The mobility of the cranial bones
5. The arbitrary mobility of the sacrum between the ilia

We do not want to present these five components of craniosacral therapy in detail here, but instead refer the reader to the relevant literature. Nevertheless, for the sake of a thorough understanding, we must describe a few aspects more precisely.

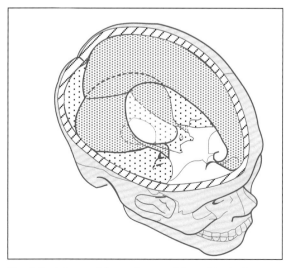

Fig. 4.2   Intracranial membranes: falx and tentorium.

The mobility of the nervous system and the fluctuation of the liquor are most likely at least partly responsible for movements of the craniosacral system, that is, they serve as a sort of motion. The interconnected membranes and bones, however, are of prime importance for the harmony of motion patterns.

The cranial dura mater adheres to the inside of the cranial bones with its parietal leaf and is connected with the periost via the sutures. The visceral leaf, in parts broken off from the parietal leaf, constitutes the cerebral membranes. These are arranged in such a way that they force the cranial bones to make very specific movements during a cranial impulse.

The cerebral and cerebellar falx form a vertical sickle in the sagittal plane that runs from the crista galli of the ethmoidal bone along the metopic suture, the sagittal suture, and to the internal occipital protuberance, all the way to the foramen magnum. They form a dividing wall between the cerebral hemispheres, as well as between the cerebellar hemispheres. The falx also connects the ethmoidal bone, frontal bone, both parietal bones, and the occipital bone.

The cerebellar tentorium runs from the clinoid processes along the upper edge of the petrous bone and the inside of the asterion, and then along the occiput up to the internal occipital protuberance. The cerebellar tentorium separates as it were the cerebrum from the cerebellum. The free edge of both sickles is in contact with the corpus callosum for the falx and with the diencephalons for the tentorium. The tentorium connects the sphenoidal, temporal, parietal, and occipital bones.

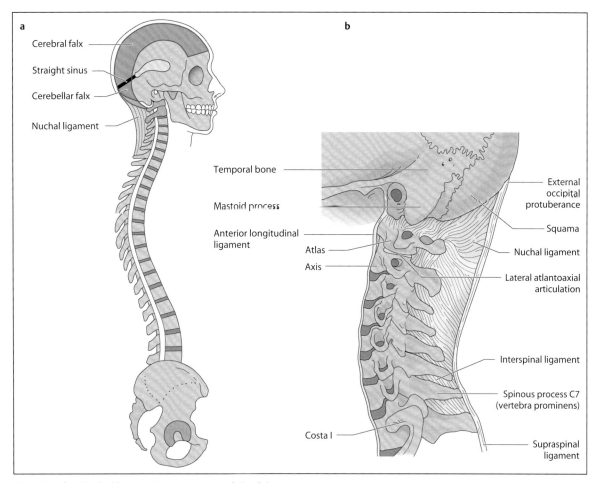

Fig. 4.3a, b Nuchal ligament as extension of the falx.

It is significant that the intracranial membranes form the venous sinuses, the venous blood conduits of the brain. Tension in these membranes can affect venous drainage from the head. The two sickles, falx, and tentorium meet in the straight sinus, also called the "Sutherland fulcrum."

The fact that the external occipital protuberance, which corresponds to the internal occipital protuberance inside the skull, serves as attachment point for the nuchal ligament on the outside of the occiput, is remarkable.

Likewise, the transverse sinus, which is formed by the cerebellar tentorium on the inside of the occiput, is located on a line with the superior nuchal line, which serves as attachment point for the trapezius muscle. The nuchal ligament is thus on the outside of the cranium the extension of the falx, and the fascia of the trapezius is the extension of the tentorium (**Figs. 4.3–4.4**).

The cerebellar falx is solidly anchored to the foramen magnum and from there passes into the spinal dura mater. Similar to the falx and tentorium, the spinal dura mater is formed by a visceral leaf, while the par-

ietal leaf passes into the periost (or rather, forms it). It hangs loose in the entire spinal cord channel and is only anchored solidly to the vertebrae at certain points. In the cranial section, it is affixed to the foramen magnum and the second cervical vertebra, and is then attached solidly in the sacral region at the level of S1/S2.

The spinal dura mater encloses the spinal cord and follows the peripheral nerves up to the intervertebral foramen, where it passes into the outer cover of the nerves. In the intervertebral foramen it is also affixed to the bone. Furthermore, there are relatively loose attachments at the vertebral bodies via the denticulate ligaments.

The dura mater is the outer envelope of the three meninges, which envelop the central nervous system. While the pia mater lies on top of the nerve mass, the arachnoid mater fills the space between the pia and dura mater, the so-called subarachnoidal space. This is filled with liquor and serves like a water bed for the brain and spinal cord.

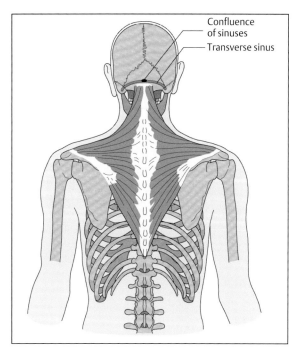

Fig. 4.4   Fascia of the trapezius as extension of the tentorium.

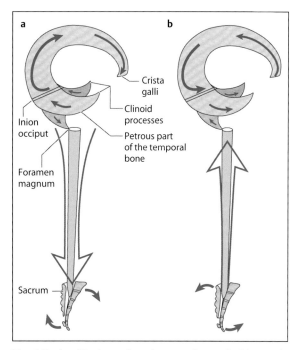

Fig. 4.5a, b   "Reciprocal tension membranes" with attachments.

The subarachnoidal space is connected to the ventricles in which the liquor is produced (choroid plexus). Some 95% of the reabsorption of the liquor takes place in the arachnoid villi of the venous sinus. The remaining 5% is reabsorbed via the lymphatic system.

The dural system is a very resistant membrane that attaches at certain places and forms a hose-like structure filled with CSF and nerves. This means that pressure or tension at one place spreads to the entire system. We can compare this to an air-filled balloon that is compromised in one spot. This pressure can be felt everywhere on the balloon. The entire dural system has five points of attachment whose common anchor is the Sutherland fulcrum:

- In front, the crista galli and clinoid processes
- Laterally, the two temporal bones
- In back, the occipital bone
- Below, the sacrum

The fact that pulling on one of these points affects all others via the Sutherland fulcrum is of clinical significance. In other words: a sacral malposition affects the occipitoatlantoaxial (OAA) complex just as much as a malposition in the temporal bone or sphenoidal bone. The consequences are even greater in the spinal column because the sensitive muscle spindles there have an exponential effect.

While the cranial sutures do not permit movement per se, as we know it from the extremities of the spinal column, they do allow for malleability. Movements related to craniosacral impulses do not cause a volume change in the cranium, but only a deformation of the entire hydraulic system including the spinal column and pelvis. Since these movements proceed harmoniously, restrictions in one point of the system manifest everywhere.

If the disturbance is significant enough, the whole system adapts in order to function. This leads to adjustments in the structures, which ultimately causes structural or postural changes. This is the meaning of the term "**reciprocal tension membranes**" (**Fig. 4.5**)

Note: Opinions differ on the trigger of craniosacral movements. In general, it is assumed that fluctuations in the liquor cause tensions in the dural system that in turn affect the bones. The special anatomy of the cranial sutures and the attachments of the dura are responsible for specific movement patterns.

4.3 The Movements and Dysfunctions of the Craniosacral Mechanism

For a detailed description, we once again refer the reader to the relevant literature. We will only describe here what is necessary for understanding the following content.

▪ Flexion and Extension

When Sutherland defined the two stages of the craniosacral rhythm, he called them flexion and extension because he considered the SBS to be the center of movement. In conforming to the nomenclature, flexion of the SBS corresponds to a reduction in the angle between the basilar part of the occiput and of the sphenoid body. Extension corresponds to an increase in this angle.

Flexion

The occipital bone makes a backward rotation, and the sphenoidal bone makes a forward rotation, in which the SBS rises. Globally, both bones make a forward movement. This is important for the relationship between occiput and atlas. **In cranial flexion, the occipital bone slides forward over the atlas (Fig. 4.6a).** This corresponds to a mechanical extension of the occiput. The ethmoidal bone, lying in front of the sphenoidal bone, makes the same rotation as the occipital bone. The paired or peripheral bones make an external rotation during flexion.

The forward movement of the occipital bone and upward movement of the basilar part shift the foramen magnum forward. This results in a cranial pull on the spinal dura mater. Consequently, the base of the sa-

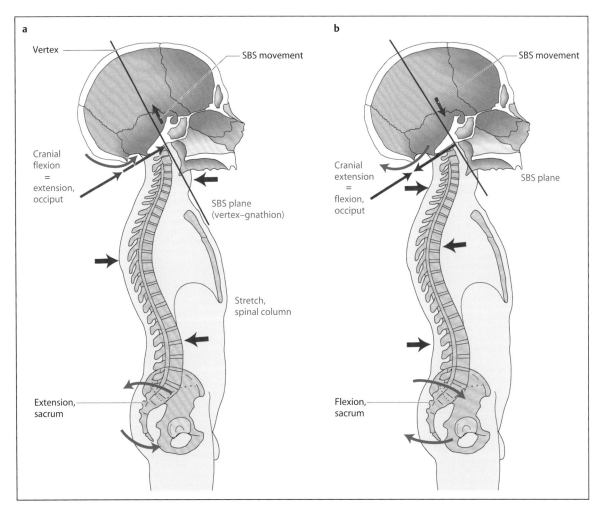

Fig. 4.6a, b **a** Biomechanics of cranial flexion: movement of the occiput over the atlas. **b** Biomechanics of cranial extension: movement of the occiput over the atlas.

crum is pulled upward, causing an extension in the sacrum and stretch in the spinal column.

Extension

Extension of the craniosacral mechanism (**Fig. 4.6b**) causes a movement in the opposite direction. The SBS drops, the occiput rotates forward, and the sphenoidal bone rotates backward. **The basilar part and the foramen magnum move backward**. From a mechanical standpoint, this corresponds to a flexion of the occiput.

The dural tube drops and the sacrum moves forward into the nutation. The ethmoid rotates forward, like the occiput. The peripheral bones make an internal rotation.

In addition to the physiological movements flexion–extension, which are induced by the organism's inherent powers, the primary respiratory mechanism (PRM), Sutherland described other movements (torsion, sidebending rotation, vertical strain, and lateral strain), which are explained in the following.

▪ Torsion

Like flexion and extension, torsion is a physiological movement. Herein, occiput and sphenoid rotate around an anteroposterior axis in the opposite direction. The movement is named according to the rotation of the sphenoidal bone (similar to the way in which the movement of the spinal column is named according to the rotation of the cranial vertebra).

Let us take a rightward rotation for an example. In this movement, the sphenoidal bone rotates to the right; the right greater wing moves upward. Because the joint face of the SBS lies not in a vertical but in a diagonal plane that stretches more or less through the vertex and gnathion, both joint partners make a movement in this diagonal plane (**Fig. 4.7**). As a result, in a torsion to the right (**Fig. 4.8**), the basilar part of the occiput moves forward and downward on the right, while the sphenoid body moves upward and backward, and in the opposite direction on the left side.

This has consequences for the occipitoatlantal (OA) joint. **On the right side, the occiput moves forward; on the left side, it moves backward. Hence the occiput stands on top of the atlas in a leftward rotation and rightward sidebending**.

Since the peripheral bones follow the movement of the central bones, we find the following in the case of a rightward rotation:

- Basilar part anterior and low on the right: right temporal in external rotation (= back right quadrant in external rotation)
- Basilar part posterior and high on the left: left temporal in internal rotation (= back left quadrant in internal rotation)
- Sphenoid body and right greater wing high: front right quadrant in external rotation
- Sphenoid body and left greater wing low: front left quadrant in internal rotation

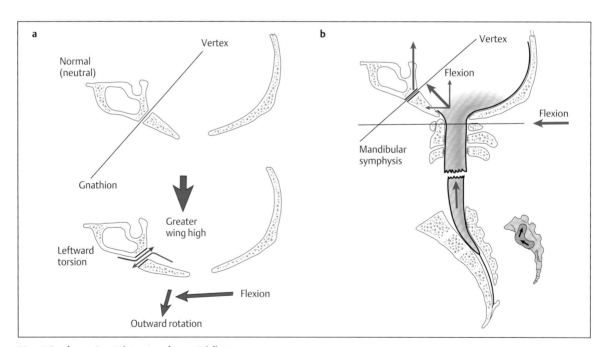

Fig. 4.7a, b a Cranial torsion, **b** cranial flexion.

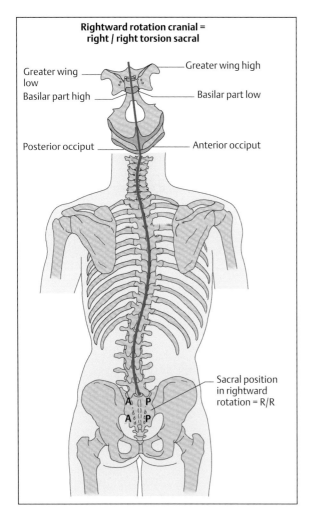

Rightward rotation cranial =
right / right torsion sacral

Greater wing low

Greater wing high

Basilar part high

Basilar part low

Posterior occiput

Anterior occiput

Sacral position in rightward rotation = R/R

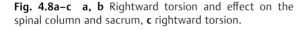

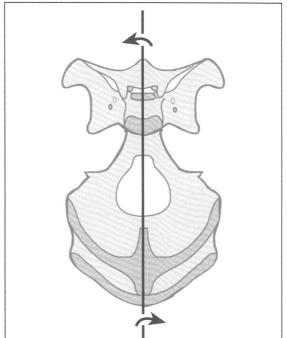

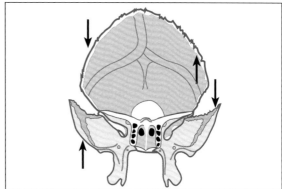

Fig. 4.8a–c a, b Rightward torsion and effect on the spinal column and sacrum, **c** rightward torsion.

Consequences for the Pelvis

In a rightward torsion of the skull, the basilar part of the occiput is in flexion on the right, that is, anterior and left posterior, that is, in extension from a craniosacral perspective. Because of this, the dura mater is pulled on the right and is relatively relaxed on the left side. This causes the base of the sacrum to drop on the left and rise on the right. This position corresponds to a rightward torsion around a right axis according to Mitchell's model.

Note: In Sutherland's times, dysfunctions of the sacrum were not named after Mitchell's model.[107, 156] The following terminology was used:

1. Sacrum in flexion
   Basis anterior–inferolateral angle (ILA) posterior
2. Sacrum in extension
   Basis posterior–ILA anterior
3. Torsion
   Basis and ILA anterior or posterior on the same side
4. Sidebending rotation
   Basis anterior and ILA posterior on one side, and the other way around on the other side. This corresponds to the sacrum anterior or posterior unilaterally.

The posterior basis of the sacrum provides for the rotation, the lower ILA for the sidebending.

■ Sidebending Rotation

According to Sutherland, the sidebending rotation is a physiological movement of the SBS as well. In this movement, the sphenoidal bone bends sideways toward the occiput—on one side—and both bones rotate together to the *same* side. This movement is named according to the side, in which the greater wing is low, for example, sidebending rotation left or sidebending rotation right (**Figs. 4.9, 4.10**).

Because of the sidebending, the sphenoid and occiput move closer together on the right side. The leftward rotation causes the sphenoidal body and basilar part to incline to the left. As a result, the top of the skull takes on a characteristic shape.

While the right side of the cranial girth is shorter and straighter, the left side becomes longer and rounder. Due to the sidebending of the SBS, "the joint opens up on the left," which affects the position of the occiput over the atlas.

On the left side, the occiput slides backward. On the right side, it is pulled forward by the sidebending. **Hence, the occiput stands in a left rotation and right sidebending over the atlas** (which restores the horizontal position).

The drop of the SBS on the left side is compensated by the right sidebending of the occiput. The peripheral cranial bones adapt as follows:
- Basilar part low on the left: left temporal in external rotation = back left cranial quadrant in external rotation
- Basilar part high on the right: right temporal in internal rotation = back right quadrant in internal rotation
- Greater wing low on the left = left right quadrant in internal rotation
- Greater wing high on the right = right front quadrant in external rotation

As the cranial bones are forced to adjust in order to harmonize, the spinal column and rest of the organism are forced to do likewise. The left rotation–right sidebending of the occiput over the atlas affects the OAA complex and the spinal dura mater as much as the lumbosacral junction. The occiput posterior on the left corresponds to an occiput in extension position on a craniosacral level.

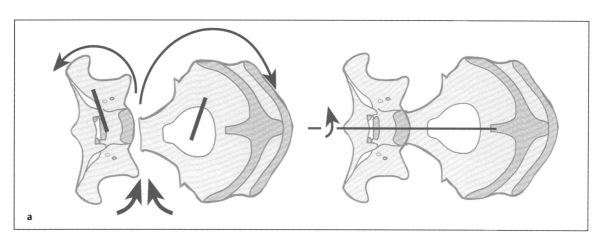

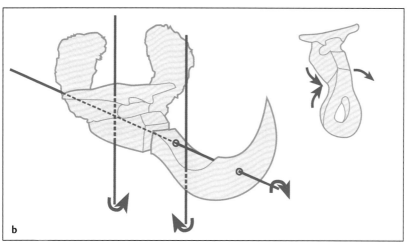

Fig. 4.9a, b Sidebending rotation to the right.

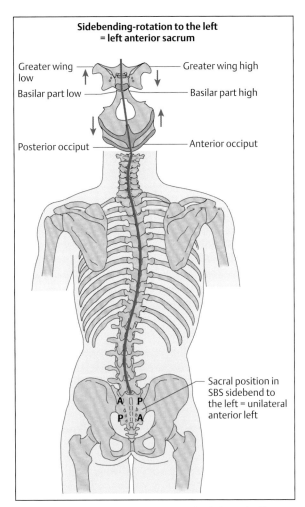

Fig. 4.10 Sidebending rotation to the left and effect on the spinal column and pelvis.

The dural tube is relaxed on the left side, as a result of which the base of the sacrum can drop forward and down on the left. On the right, the occiput is anterior, that is, in flexion position from a craniosacral viewpoint. The dural tube is tensed and the base of the cranium is kept cranial-posterior. The sacrum makes a rotation to the right. This corresponds to the rightward rotation of the occiput and sphenoid in a sidebending rotation to the left.

> *Note:* To ensure functionality, the balancing organs (comparable to a spirit level) and eyes have to be horizontal. The eyes, moreover, have to be in the same frontal plane to avoid excessive strain on the eye muscles. The ideal adjustment zone for this purpose is in the OAA joints.

■ Vertical Strain and Lateral Strain

In addition to the four physiological movements described above the SBS also executes so-called aphysiological movements.

In vertical strain, the SBS is shifted caudally in the cranium. The sphenoidal body shifts upward or downward in relation to the basilar part of the occiput. The facial skull, spinal column, and pelvis are affected correspondingly (flexion–external rotation or extension–internal rotation position).

In lateral strain, the occiput and sphenoid shift in a horizontal plane. This does not lead to obvious changes in the spinal column. This strain is most commonly found in combination with other cranial dysfunctions, such as flexion, extension, torsion, or sidebending rotation. It is frequently traumatic in nature or the result of persistent tensions in the areas influenced by the sphenoid or occiput:

- Falling on the buttocks, getting hit on the back of the head, or tensions in the spinal dural mater all put strain on the occiput.
- Facial traumas or persistent ventral fascial pull, on the other hand, affect the sphenoidal bone and cause strain in the sphenoidal bone.

■ Compression Dysfunction in the Sphenobasilar Synchondrosis

A compression dysfunction has no significant effect on the spinal column or other cranial bones in the sense of provoking malposture. It only has extremely negative results for the mechanics of the PRM and therefore must be given primary attention in treatment when it occurs. It involves a traumatic lesion in which the movements of the occiput and sphenoid are clearly limited.

It can be caused by a fall on the buttocks or a hit on the occiput, glabella, or nasion. Compressions often arise during birth when the head becomes stuck in the birth canal and the baby is thereby exposed to pressure during contractions.

■ Intraossal Dysfunction

Intraossal Lesions of the Cranial Bones

Because the bones grow from the ossification points out into the periphery, compression of the sutures is the most likely cause of intraossal lesions in the cranial bones. Tensions in the cranial membranes can also be a cause.

Intrauterine and perinatal factors are mainly responsible for a compression of the sutures. It is obvious that these lesions, as we view them from the osteopathic perspective, only arise during the developing years.

Intraossal Lesions of the Skull Base

As with the bones in the extremities, trauma, compression, or persistent tension in the growth sutures can also lead to deformation in the cranial bones. This is particularly dramatic when the sphenoidal, temporal, occipital, or sacral bones are affected.

All of these bones consist at birth of several parts that are only fused together completely by the age of 8–12 years. Deformation in these bones can result in malposition of the SBS and the craniocervical junction, thereby affecting the locomotor system.

Intraossal lesions in these bones can cause specific damage in certain areas of the body:

- Lesions between the presphenoid and postsphenoid affect the facial skull (especially the eyes).
- Lesions in the temporal bone can negatively affect hearing, the organs of equilibrium, and the temporomandibular joint.
- Intraossal lesions in the sacrum can have a negative impact on the postural and motion functions of the spinal column and lower extremities.
- The most far-reaching effect, not only on posture, is most likely caused by lesions in the occipitoatlantal region.
- According to Sutherland, deformations in the area of the basilar part and condylar part are responsible for a number of complaints[101, 102]:
  - Disorders in the cranial nerves VI–XII due to compression around the foramina or tension of the membranes. We must not forget that the dura mater accompanies the cranial nerves up to the foramina and is anchored securely there.
  - Impaired circulation: 95% of the venous blood leaves the head via the jugular foramina. Shifts in the condylar or basilar parts can change these openings. On the other hand, malpositions of the cranial basis can cause SBS lesions that lead to tension in the membranes. As a result, the venous sinuses are affected, which can in turn influence circulation in the brain. We must not forget that the dura mater accompanies the cranial nerves up to the foramina and is anchored securely there.
  - A change in the lumina of the foramen magnum can exert pressure on the brain stem and thereby cause a number of effects. The medulla and pons lie on top of the basilar part of the occiput and the SBS. Damage to the pyramidal tracts is a common cause of spastic states in cerebral palsy. Malpositions in the region of the basilar part can be involved in this.

Note: For nerve function to be disturbed, the nerve mass must not necessarily be compromised. Disturbed vascular supply is enough. Pressure or membranous tensions are able to irritate the vessels that supply the nerves.

As we mentioned earlier, tensions in one part of the cerebral membranes are transferred to the entire dural system. Because the dura mater is anchored solidly to the foramen magnum and S2, deformations in these areas have consequences for the entire postural system. For this reason, we are going to take a closer look at intraossal lesions in the occiput.

Intraossal Lesions in the Occiput

We need to point out once more that cranial base originates from cartilage, while the arch is made from membranes. The roof is therefore more adaptable than the base.

During birth and in early childhood, the membranes are more resistant than the bones. The membranes hold together the bones that consist of several parts. Perinatal trauma or tension, as well as accidents in infancy, can therefore affect the growth sutures of the bones and immediately or later manifest during growth spurts (scoliosis, kypholordosis, cross-bite, and so on).

At birth, the occiput consists of four parts (**Fig. 4.11a**) that are held together by the dura mater and the pericranium:

1. Squamous part of the occipital bone
2. and 3. The two lateral masses or condylar parts
4. Basilar part

These four parts form the frame of the foramen magnum.

The two occipital condyles are not yet fully developed at birth and consist of two-thirds of the condylar part and one-third of the basilar part. The atlas also consists of several parts (**Fig 4.11b**).

In contrast to the occiput, the facets are formed earlier. In addition, the atlas arches are stabilized by the strong transverse ligament of the atlas. As a result, the occiput condyles and the foramen magnum are more likely to suffer from deformations than the atlas. It is also significant that the occiput condyles and atlas facets are oriented medially forward.

The longitudinal axes of both joints converge in the front in a point below the SBS. They form an angle of ± 30º with each other. Forced flexion and extension movements can result in compression of the growth sutures because the condyles "threaten to derail." Most common is the deformation of the cranial base during the birth process.

During a normal natural birth, the head of the newborn is compromised during the passage through the birth canal according to a certain pattern. In addition, a rotation and flexion–extension movement occurs in the cervical spinal column. If for any reason the birth canal is too narrow for the child's head, the mother's contractions can exert such pressure on the cervico-occipital junction that the weakest structures give in. Depending on the condition of the head at the time, the forces focus on a certain point, which causes a characteristic lesion there.

Compression in the sagittal plane (symmetrical pressure on the supraocciput) can press the condyles forward too strongly. This can change the position of the condylar parts.

The lumen of the foramen magnum, as well as that of the jugular foramina, may become reduced. This can result in compression of the sutures between the occiput and the temporal bone. The pressure can also shift the basilar part. As a result, vertical strains (a caudal shift of the basilar part) can arise.

The therapist can palpate this position from the shape of the supraocciput and the position of the inion, among other things. Under diagonal pressure on the occiput, when the baby's head is in a rotated position above the atlas, it can happen that a condyle is pushed forward. This condyle is then shifted forward medially and the condyle on the other side is shifted laterally. As a result, we may see torsions, sidebending rotation, or lateral strains (a shift of the basilar part to lateral) in the SBS.

The foramen magnum and jugular foramina can change. The sutures between the occiput and the temporal bone can become compromised. The therapist can recognize this malposition from the relation between the occiput and the lateral mass of the atlas, as well as by comparing the nuchal (or supraoccipital) line on the left and right side. In both cases, the posture of the spinal column and the muscle tone are affected:

- The position of the condyles influences the tension of the dural tube up to the sacrum as well as forward up to the crista galli.
- Symmetrical malpositions are felt as an increased flexed or extended posture.
- Asymmetrical positions of the occiput condyles lead to twisting of the dural tube, with a resulting pelvic twist.

Fig. 4.11a, b   **a** Occipital bone, **b** atlas and axis in a newborn.

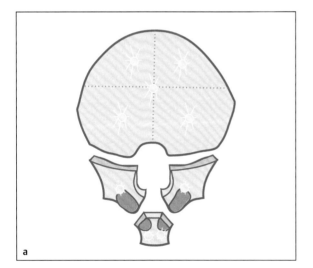

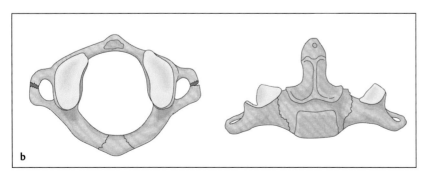

- The suboccipital muscles are particularly important for muscle tone.
- The great sensitivity of the muscle spindles as well as the extremely rich supply of the short neck muscles with muscle spindles in the suboccipital area are responsible for the fact that this area is so significant for regulating muscle tension in general and posture in particular.

Notes:

- Posturologists were able to demonstrate with experiments, in which the distribution of weight to both feet was measured, that a manipulation of C2, the relaxation of the falx, and the treatment of the temporomandibular joint results in obvious improvement in the distribution of weight.[153, 154] All osteopaths should be familiar with the connection between these three structures and the short neck muscles.
- In microscopic examinations of the short neck muscles, it was proven that they contain ± 6 times as many muscle spindles as the gluteal musculature (per cm³ of muscle mass).
- Viola Frymann was able to show with a substantial collection of skulls that deformations of the skull basis are common and that malpositions and malformations of the condyles and changes in the foramen magnum, jugular foramina, and hypoglossal canal commonly occur together.[57] In most cases, these are accompanied by asymmetries in the cranial vault. When cranial scoliosis is visible, parietal scoliosis is also present. How pronounced it is depends on the adaptive capabilities of the organism.
- The research results of I. Korr and M. Patterson strongly suggest that longer-lasting myofascial tensions and imbalances cause structural changes.[79, 112]
- It is also an interesting fact that the clivus and the SBS plane have the same vertical inclination as the longitudinal axis and the promontorium of the sacrum.

■ Sacral Dysfunctions

Dysfunctions of the sacrum are affected via the spinal dura mater, the "core link," in the craniosacral mechanism:

Sacral nutation	cranial extension
Sacral contranutation	cranial flexion
Sacral torsion	SBS torsion
Unilateral sacral flexion	sidebending rotation

The cause of sacral dysfunctions can be found in traumas, persistent malposture, or lumbar spinal column (LSC) dysfunctions or visceral disorders. We should not forget here that infants frequently fall on their buttocks.

If we develop this notion of the asymmetry of membranous tensions and corresponding muscular imbalances further, we can conclude that this problem can easily serve as an explanation for scoliosis and other asymmetries, when left untreated.

Some authors, among them Harold Magoun, posit that asymmetrical dural tension can have a negative effect on growth. It appears that differences in leg length that occur in children and youths do not disappear completely in adults.[145] When we take into consideration the fact that nerves transport not only nerve impulses but also molecules that are vital for the nutrition of the supplied structures, we can see how fascial or membranous tensions can easily affect the nutrition of tissue during growth spurts in such a way that it causes asymmetries.

> We can only conclude from the above that newborns should be examined and if necessary treated osteopathically to ensure the best possible harmonious development.

4.4   The Influence of Cranial Dysfunctions and Malpostures on the Periphery

Craniosacral dysfunctions afflict not only the axial skeleton, but also the extremities. Even the visceral region is affected.

Sutherland was an all-around outstanding osteopath. He integrated Still's way of thinking like nobody else and was an excellent observer on top of that. Because of his keen sense of observation and palpation and his love for experimenting, he managed not only to decode the craniosacral mechanism, but he also realized the impact of this craniosacral mechanism on the

entire body. Hence, he realized that the entire organism acts analogously to the craniosacral mechanism.

During thoracic inhalation, the skull expands like in the cranial flexion stage, while expiration results in a movement like in the extension stage. Sutherland likewise realized that the entire body makes an external rotation during thoracic inhalation and cranial flexion, and an internal rotation during the opposite stage. He concluded from this that there are two movement patterns:

- A flexion pattern, associated with external rotation and abduction
- An extension pattern, associated with internal rotation and adduction

We can easily comprehend this with a simple experiment. Compare an inspiration in which arms and legs are fully rotated inward, with one in which the arms and legs are fully rotated outward. The inspiration is much deeper when the extremities are rotated outward.

For the description of the muscle chains (see Chapter 8, p. 77), we have adopted Sutherland's model. We are convinced that there are two myofascial chains in each half of the body:

- A flexion chain
- An extension chain

When the extension chain dominates bilaterally, the spinal column is stretched while head and extremities are in flexion, external rotation (and abduction for the extremities). When the flexion chain dominates, this increases the curvature in the spinal column, the extremities and the cranium are in extension, internal rotation (and adduction for the extremities). In the case of asymmetrical dominance, one half of the body acts according to the flexion pattern, while the other acts according to the extension pattern.

In Chapter 8, we describe in detail how bones and joints act in the case of dominance of one chain. We can thereby understand the possible dysfunctions that result from this.

Dominant muscle chains can be triggered in the extremities as well as in the organs or cranial basis. In each case, however, we find a certain SBS position, a position of the OAA complex that corresponds to this position, and a certain position of the lumbosacral junction (LSJ).

5 The Biomechanical Model of John Martin Littlejohn—The Mechanics of the Spine

5.1 History

John Martin Littlejohn emigrated from Great Britain to the United States in 1892 for health reasons. He suffered from a supposedly incurable neck disorder. Upon his arrival, he heard of the unbelievable treatment outcomes of a Dr. Still and decided to look him up.

Still was not only able to relieve Littlejohn of his suffering, but managed to arouse his interest in osteopathy to such an extent that Littlejohn stayed in Kirksville for training. He remained with Still for several years, acting as docent and dean at the American School of Osteopathy. At the beginning of the 20th century, he founded the American College of Osteopathy and Surgery in Chicago with his two brothers.

After he graduated from medical school in Chicago and received a doctorate, he returned to England. In 1917, he founded the British School of Osteopathy in London. John Martin Littlejohn is not the first osteopath who came from the United States to Europe. Several others had come to Great Britain before him and founded the British Osteopathy Association there in 1911. These were Dunham, Willard-Walker, and Horn. Nevertheless, we can claim that Littlejohn brought osteopathy to Europe. It was, after all, his theories about the biomechanics of the spine that shaped British (and European) osteopathy for decades.

Littlejohn is regarded in osteopathy simply as *the mechanic*. It is true that his perspective on the func-

tions of the spine is very mechanical, but nevertheless, functionality and globality are just as central for him. In his view, the spine (and the locomotor system) is a unit that is subject to certain mechanical laws. Thus, the spine is, for example, constantly affected by gravity. In addition, the individual spine segments do not act in isolation, but the entire trunk reacts as a unit to external and internal influences.

Like all osteopaths, he realized that in different patients we find constantly recurring identical patterns, identical regions in dysfunction, and often, identical symptoms. This led him to search for a mechanical explanation for these patterns. We must note here that in his early years, nothing was known of cranial osteopathy or visceral osteopathy, as we know them today in Europe.

Both Still and Littlejohn were convinced that the spine plays a key role in the formation and treatment of disease. The enthusiastic physiologist Littlejohn used physical laws to help him explain the biomechanics of the spine. In his work *The Mechanics of the Spine*, he introduces an interesting model of thinking in which force lines, pivots, spine curvatures, curves, and arches provide explanations for dysfunctions and postural patterns[97].

5.2 The "Mechanics of the Spine" and the Force Lines of the Body

Compressive and tensile forces play an important role in physics. The same holds true in human physiology. Cell metabolism depends on pressure conditions (see the formation of arthritis, supply of intervertebral disks and cartilage, and so on). Kapandji[74] writes about the significance of spinal column curvatures for its stability ($R = N^2 + 1$; R = resistance; N = number of curvatures). There is another physical law that states that an arch that is bent to one side has the tendency to rotate with the convex side into the newly formed convexity (see neutral position–sidebending–rotation [NSR] in Chapter 3).

Note: It is an interesting fact that that the trunk consists of two cavities that both exert an expansive force.

Both the lungs and the intestines contain air and have a tendency to expand. The thorax and the abdominal cavity are surrounded by muscles that exert force toward the inside.

Muscles have the characteristic that they maintain the same basic tone in every position. Under normal conditions, the two forces neutralize each other. This phenomenon is comparable to the dural tube that is turned into a water column by the liquor and functions as a unit. The entire trunk acts as a unit.

Littlejohn described six force lines with which he tried to explain the behavior of the spine under the strain of gravity, as well as the formation of dysfunctions in constantly recurring patterns:

▪ The Central Gravity Line

In reality, this refers to two lines: a left and a right. Its course is as follows (**Fig. 5.1**):
- ± 1 cm behind the sella turcica
- ± 1 cm in front of the atlas facets
- Through the middle of the transverse muscles C3–C6
- In front of the vertebral body of T4
- Through the costovertebral joints K2–K10
- Through the vertebral body of L3
- At the level of L3, the two lines divide, to run through the legs to the center of the foot

These are mobile lines that are able to change their course to adapt to posture.

▪ The Anterior Body Line

It is parallel to the central gravity line and runs from the symphysis menti to the pubic symphysis (**Fig. 5.2**). Its course depends on pressure conditions in the thorax and abdomen. Hence, it gives clues about the correlation between posture and the pressure conditions in the cavities. When the postural equilibrium changes, pressure conditions in the abdominal and thoracic cavities adjust. Increased pressure in the abdomen, for example, changes the course of the anterior body line and thereby also that of the central gravity line.

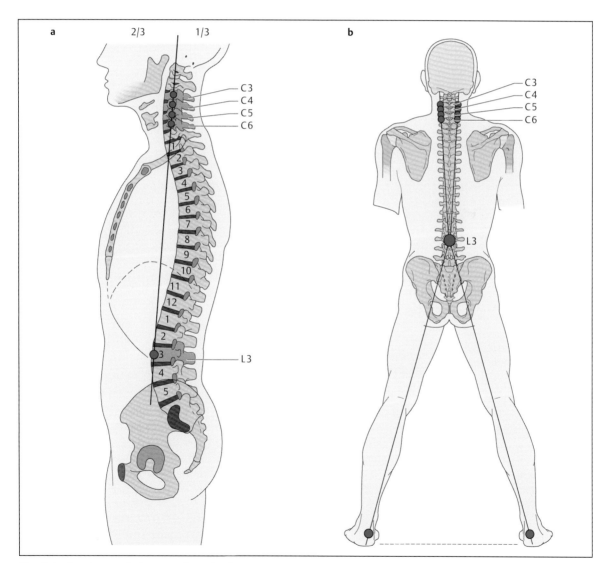

Fig. 5.1a, b Course of the central gravity line.

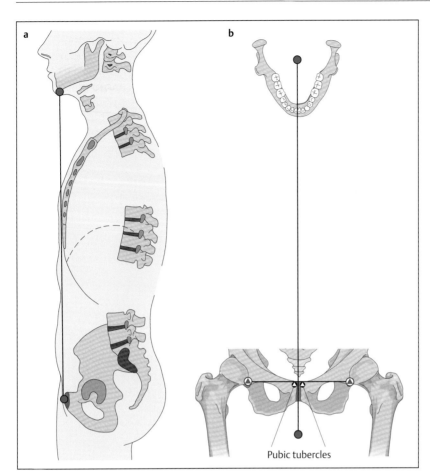

Fig. 5.2a, b Course of the anterior body line.

Because the diaphragms are important for the balance of pressure in the cavities, the anterior body line is in close contact with them. The tension of the abdominal wall is related to the tension of the thoracic diaphragm. The following two scenarios can occur (**Fig. 5.3a, b**):

The Anterior Body Line Falls in Front of the Pubic Symphysis

* Increased pressure on the abdominal wall
* Growing tension on the inguinal ligament, which can lead to hernias
* Increased cervical spinal column (CSC) lordosis
* The chin is stretched forward and up.
* Tensions in the cervicothoracic, thoracolumbar, and lumbosacral junctions (CTJ, TLJ, LSJ)
* Recurvatum in the knee
* Susceptibility to otorhinolaryngology (ORL) disorders

The Anterior Body Line Falls Behind the Pubic Symphysis

* Abdominal pressure shifts backward onto the lower abdominal organs and the aorta and iliac vessels.
* The CSC is stretched and the chin is pulled in.
* Thoracic spinal column (TSC) kyphosis and tension between the shoulder blades
* Hanging shoulders
* Tendency to lumbar hyperlordosis
* Flat thorax
* Tendency to organ prolapse
* Tensions in the iliosacral joint (ISJ) area
* Flexum of the knee
* Pull on the ischiocrural musculature
* Weight shift onto the heels

■ The Anteroposterior Line

This line begins in the opisthion, runs through the anterior tubercle of the atlas, through the vertebral bodies T11 and T12, and through the arch joints of L4–L5, and traverses S1, to end at the tip of the coccyx.

This line makes a unit of the entire spine and turns T11 and T12 into key vertebrae for anteroposterior balance and trunk torsions. Asymmetrical strain on the arms or legs, trunk torsions, or straightening the spine place a burden on T11 and T12. These vertebrae also play a role in the circulation of the abdomen.

Two Posteroanterior Lines

Both lines run along the back edge of the foramen magnum through the second ribs and pass through the vertebral bodies L2 and L3, to end in the hip joints. Like the anteroposterior line, they run in front of T4.

Both lines connect the occipitoatlantal (OA) joints with the second ribs and T2, and thereby guarantee even tension in the CSC. They direct the pressure conditions to the hip joints when standing and to the protuberances when sitting. The main function of these lines lies in maintaining an optimal tension relation between neck, trunk, and legs on the one hand, and abdomen and thorax on the other.

The anteroposterior line and the two posteroanterior lines form the so-called force polygon (**Fig. 5.4**).

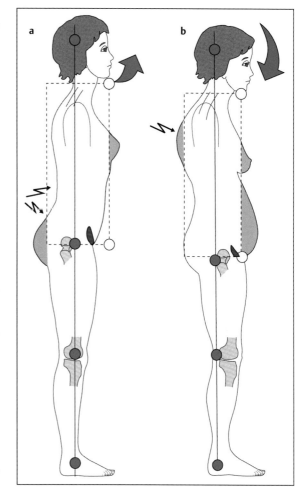

Fig. 5.3a, b Anteroposterior shift of the anterior body line.

5.3 The Force Polygon

Littlejohn's force polygon (**Fig. 5.5**) consists of two triangular pyramids whose tips attach in front of the vertebral body of T4. The two posteroanterior lines and the anteroposterior line balance each other out and cross in front of T4. The result of these three lines is the central gravity line that runs through L3.

The lower pyramid has a solid base, consisting of the hip joints and the coccyx. The foramen magnum serves as the base of the upper pyramid. It is stabilized by myofascial structures. Pelvic dysfunctions and occipitoatlantoaxial (OAA) lesions influence T3–T4. When walking, both pyramids turn in opposite directions. We can see this from the opposite arm and leg movements.

When the stance leg is on the left and the swing leg on the right, the lower pyramid forms a convexity with rightward rotation, while the upper pyramid makes a convexity with leftward rotation. The central gravity line connects L3 with the hip joints.

The anteroposterior line connects the atlas and the coccyx, running through L3. This creates a third pyramid, which also has the pelvis as a solid base and L3 as its tip.

All three pyramids depend on the pressure conditions in the cavities, the two lower ones directly and the upper pyramid indirectly through myofascial tensions.

Inhalation and exhalation not only change the pressure in the thorax and abdomen, but also cause the spine to stretch during inhalation.

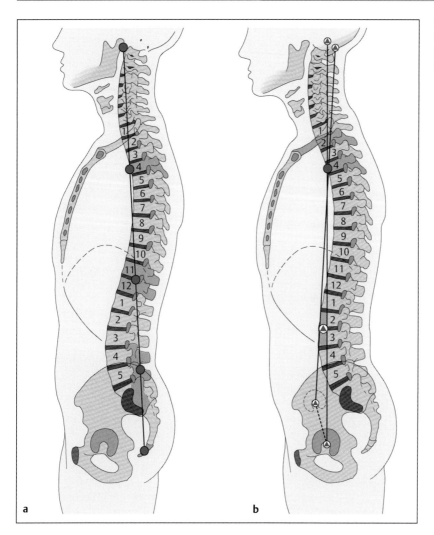

Fig. 5.4a, b Course of the anteroposterior line and the two posteroanterior lines, which constitute the force polygon.

a

b

5.4   Arches, Pivots, and Double Arches (Fig. 5.6)

Arches

From an anatomical perspective, the spine consists of four arches:
- Cervical: atlas–T1
- Thoracic: T2–T12
- Lumbar: L1–L5
- Sacral: sacrum–coccyx

Littlejohn also divided the spine into four arches, but from a functional perspective. He defined the arches as areas of the spine between so-called pivots. The arches move as a whole. The functional arches are as follows:
- Upper arch: C1–C4
- Middle arch: C6–T8
- Lower arch: T10–L4
- Sacrum

This classification into functional arches makes it possible to demonstrate how the individual spinal segments relate to each other. By accepting Littlejohn's model of force lines and his understanding of the effect of individual muscle groups as well as of the anatomical characteristics of individual vertebrae, we can then accept certain vertebrae as pivots.

■ Pivots

There are anatomical, physiological, and functional pivots.

Anatomical pivots are the atypical vertebrae. They force segments of the spine to behave in specific ways due to their special anatomical shape. Anatomical pivots are: C2–L5–sacrum.

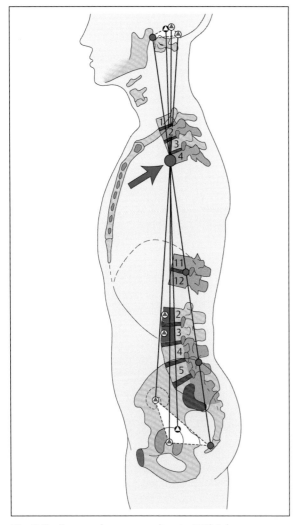

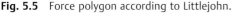

Fig. 5.5 Force polygon according to Littlejohn.

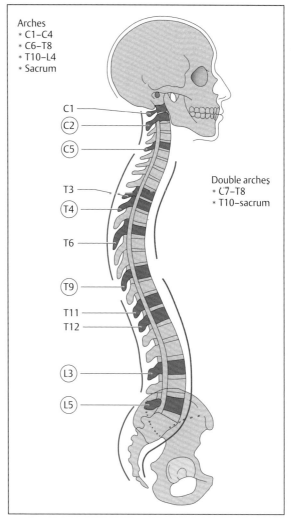

Fig. 5.6 Arches, double arches, and pivot vertebrae.

Littlejohn associated the atlas with the head and therefore did not consider it as a pivot.

Physiological pivots are located in between curvatures, that is, where a lordosis transitions into a kyphosis: C5–T9–L5.

Functional pivots are vertebrae that gain special significance because of their mechanical function. These are: C2/T4/L3:

- C2 is a pivot for the head. The extremely sensitive suboccipital musculature connects the OAA complex.
- T4 is a pivot because the head rotation reaches to T4–T5. In addition, T4 is an important intersection for Littlejohn's force lines.
- L3 is the lowest lumbar vertebra that is not directly connected by ligaments to the pelvis.

Because of their connection through the iliolumbar ligaments, L4 and L5 belong to the pelvis (similar to the connection of C1 and C2 to the head). In addition, L3 is the gravitational center of the whole body for Suther-

land. Dysfunctions of these pivot vertebrae are extremely common. Only in very rare cases are they manipulated in isolation. The associated arches should always be treated in conjunction.

Double Arches

Littlejohn described two double arches:
- The upper posterior arch: C7–T8
- The lower anterior arch: T10–sacrum

From a mechanical perspective, it is interesting to note that the upper posterior arch carries the weight of the head, thorax, and upper extremities and shifts it dorsally, so that it is then counterbalanced by the lower anterior arch and directed towards the hips.

The apex of the double arches is located for the upper arch at the level of T4–T5, and for the lower arch at the level of L2–L3. Both of these segments are very susceptible to dysfunctions. For Littlejohn, the following were weak points in this system: C7, fifth rib, T9, T11, T12, L2, L3:

- C7 is located at the transition between a mobile and a rigid spinal segment.
- T9 is a functional pivot between two arches and between an anterior and posterior double arch.
- T11 and T12 are the torsion center of the spine.
- The fifth rib is located in the transition zone between the upper thorax and the CSC and the lower thorax and the LSC.
- L2 and L3 are the weakest point in the entire spine because the weight of the whole body manifests here: the weight of the trunk presses from above and the lower extremities pull downward during walking.

In the case of postural imbalances, compensative actions tend to organize around these weak points in the spine.

Littlejohn, and later also his students John Wernham and T.E. Hall, describe in their writings the relationships between the organs, the neurovegetative system, and the endocrine system. Furthermore, he explains and substantiates his therapeutic procedures. For obvious reasons, we had to limit ourselves here to reviewing those aspects that fit into the context of this book.

A further development of this model has led to an interesting osteopathic treatment method, namely SAT (specific adjustment technique). We present this method in the following section.

5.5 Specific Adjustment Technique According to Dummer[53, 88]

■ History

The invention of specific adjustment technique (SAT) was most likely coincidental. During a flu epidemic in the 1950s, the osteopath and chiropractor Parnall Bradbury happened to be the only therapist on call in his clinic. Because of the enormous number of patients in need of treatment, Bradbury had only limited time for each treatment. Thus, he decided to only manipulate the most conspicuous segment in each patient.

His success was so great that he further analyzed this method. Particularly effective were those treatments in which he manipulated the atypical vertebrae. Parnall Bradbury was Littlejohn's student and was therefore familiar with his model of force lines. In his chiropractic training, he had learned the "whole-in-one

manipulation of the upper CSC." Incidentally, the treatment of one segment, of the key lesion, followed Still's principle to "find it, fix it, and leave it alone."

Together with the physician Dudley Tee, he completed a series of investigations to analyze the effectiveness of manipulating key lesions and introduced this method in his book *Spinology*. Herein, he defined the term for "positional lesions." This refers mostly to traumatic blockages of atypical vertebrae, such as in whiplash injuries. According to Bradbury, this vertebra has to be repositioned with an impulse technique, in which the impulse is exactly opposite the force vector that caused the blockage. This method was developed further and refined by Bradbury's student Tom Dummer. It is not only applied in traumatic lesions.

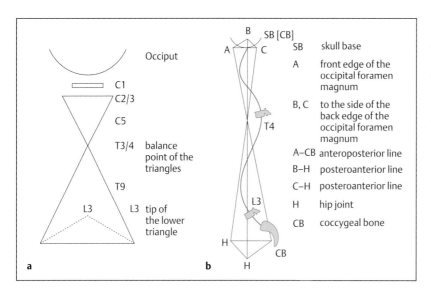

Occiput

C1
C2/3
C5
T3/4 balance point of the triangles
T9
L3   L3 tip of the lower triangle

a

B SB [CB]
A   C
T4
L3
H
CB
H

b

SB	skull base
A	front edge of the occipital foramen magnum
B, C	to the side of the back edge of the occipital foramen magnum
A–CB	anteroposterior line
B–H	posteroanterior line
C–H	posteroanterior line
H	hip joint
CB	coccygeal bone

Fig. 5.7a, b a Littlejohn's model. Inter-curve pivots are C5, T9, and L5, atypical vertebrae are C1, C2, and L5/S1. **b** Polygon of forces according to Littlejohn, demonstrating the mechanical relations and functions of the spine.

Depending on the localization of the "primary lesion" (cervical or sacral), the therapist follows a certain order in the manipulation of key segments, manipulating only one segment in each treatment.

▪ Procedure

The therapist searches for the key segment in need of treatment by dividing the locomotor system into three units. For each unit, a number of specific tests exist. The goal is to find the dominating unit.

In each unit, there are certain vertebrae that are particularly significant. These are the so-called pivots from Littlejohn's model (**Fig. 5.7**): C1, C2, C3, C5, T3, T4, T9, T11, T12, L3, L5, sacrum.

Note:
- Different pivots are affected, depending on whether it is a traumatic or adaptive case.
- Opinions differ on whether the pivot vertebrae should be manipulated or not.

A pivot is always a turning point for a group of vertebrae. Therefore, it is always recommended to also treat this group of vertebrae, for which gentle techniques are more appropriate.

▪ The Three Units

Dividing the organism into three units is, according to Littlejohn's model, very logical and practical because it makes sense neurologically as well as mechanically. The three units derive from the three pyramids of the force polygon:

Unit 1

Lower extremities, pelvis, and lower LSC from L3 down.

This unit is related to locomotion.

Unit 2

Cranium, CSC, upper TSC up to T4, shoulders and arms, upper thorax.

Vegetative functions of the head, throat, and thorax.

Unit 3

Lower thorax, vertebrae T4–L3.

Vegetative functions of the abdomen.

Note: It is interesting to observe that these three units are basically equivalent to the three lower hinge areas of Zink's model. Littlejohn's model lacks the cervicooccipital junction as an isolated unit. Instead, it is considered as Unit 2 together with the CTJ. Nevertheless, because of its special characteristics (atypical vertebra, parasympathicus area), it can, in our opinion, also be considered as a separate unit, with special significance for the craniosacral system.

6 Postural Muscles, Phasic Muscles, and Crossed Syndrome (Vladimir Janda's Contribution to Myofascial Treatment Methods[40, 41, 86, 87, 107])

In addition to other functions, the locomotor system has two important tasks:

- Stability = posture
- Mobility = motorics, movement

6.1 Posture

Maintaining balance is one of the greatest functions of the locomotor system. To fulfill this task, the organism collects a large amount of information from receptors in the entire organism. In addition to the equilibrium organs, the proprioceptors in the muscles, tendons, fasciae, and joints play a significant role. The eyes and ears are important as well. Less well-known is the fact that the temporomandibular joint and the organs influence the muscles and therefore indirectly also the posture and motorics of the body.

6.2 Motorics

The bodily function of motorics serves to satisfy our basic human needs. It is carried out by muscles. Optimal muscular activity requires good balance as well as coordination between the individual groups of muscles (inhibition of antagonists, coactivation of synergists). Both functions are directed by the central nervous system. This process involves specific posture and movement patterns that were acquired in the course of ontogenesis. These are also called motoric stereotypes or motion patterns. Examples include a person's characteristic gait or posture. Disturbed balance between individual groups of muscles, that is, deviations from optimal motion patterns, frequently develop in early childhood (many are probably of perinatal origin).

Micro- and macro-traumas as well as general habits contribute to the formation of motion patterns. Disturbed posture, as well as uncoordinated patterns, lead to muscular imbalances with excessive strain. Any disturbed function in the joints is reflected in muscular tensions. This in turn impairs postural and movement patterns.

Pain plays a key role here. The pain threshold determines whether a disturbance of joint function manifests as disease. As soon as this is the case, the entire locomotor system attempts to adapt and compensate to make the state bearable and maintain the organism's functionality.

Research has demonstrated that in cases of spastic paralysis, muscles have been inhibited even though they have not been paralyzed. The same phenomenon occurs in trigger points. Pain causes a weakening of the muscle. This promotes malpositions.

The Czech physician Vladimir Janda carried out interesting research in the area of manual medicine and specifically in the area of muscle functions. Some of his observations are important for the treatment of dysfunctions in the locomotor system. He discovered, for example, that **patients with poor motoric stereotypes and muscular imbalances also showed neurological deficits**. Movements were poorly coordinated and awkward. Impaired sensitivity, especially in the proprioceptors, as well as poor adaptation to stressful situations, caused uncontrolled behavior. Janda found these signs in children as well as adults, with the exception that adults additionally suffered from disturbed vertebral functions and pain.

Knowing motoric stereotypes and the function of individual muscles in the interplay of muscle groups allows the therapist to influence pathological patterns more accurately.

Example: Quadriceps and ischiocrural muscles are antagonists in knee stretching and movements, but synergists in stabilizing the knee during walking. During walking, foot lifters, knee benders, and hip flexors all cooperate synergistically. The synergy of muscle activities is even more obvious in pathological states. It is more important to observe a muscle in the framework of the entire motion pattern than in isolation.

6.3   Skeletal Muscle Fiber Types

Another important finding of Janda's is the fact that the behavior of weakened and shortened (contracted) muscle groups is not subject to coincidence but to certain laws.

Microscopic and electrophysiological investigations have demonstrated the existence of two different types of cross-striped muscle fibers from a functional perspective: red and white. Both types of muscle fibers are found in all muscles, but in varying quantities. The behavior of muscles is influenced by the amount of muscle fibers of a particular type. First, we describe the characteristics of both types of muscle fibers.

Postural Muscle Fibers (Red Fibers): Type I Fibers (Slow-twitch Fibers)

- Diameter of ± 50 mm
- High content of myoglobin (red color)
- Thick z disks
- High number of mitochondria
- High amount of neutral fat
- Oxidative metabolism predominates
- Low glycogenolytic and glycolytic activity
- High mitochondrial enzyme activity
- Slow contraction speed
- Suited for endurance and support functions
- Tendency to shorten
- Treatment: stretching

Phasic Muscle Fibers (White Fibers): Type II Fibers (Fast-twitch Fibers)

- Diameter of 80–100 mm
- Strongly developed sarcoplasmic reticulum
- Thin z disks
- Contain less mitochondria, lipids, and glycogen
- High myosin and actomyosin ATPase activity
- Anaerobic metabolism dominates
- High glycogen consumption
- Serves for quick short efforts
- Additional strength is caused by increased impulse frequency
- Tendency to weaken
- Treatment: strengthening

Muscles that contain primarily red muscle fibers tend towards hyperactivity, tension, shortening, and hypertonicity. Muscles that contain more white fibers tend to weaken and slacken instead.

There are controversial names for the two muscle types. We use Janda's terminology, calling muscles that contain primarily red fibers **postural muscles** and those that contain primarily white fibers **phasic muscles** (**Fig. 6.1**).

In his research, Janda was able to find that in most people, certain muscles always have a tendency to shorten and others have a tendency to weaken:

Muscles with a Tendency to Shorten

- Short extensors of the head joints
- Levator scapula
- Middle and upper section of the trapezius
- Lumbar section of the erector spinae
- Quadratus lumborum
- Muscles of mastication
- Sternocleidomastoideus (SCM)
- Scalene muscles
- Subscapularis
- Pectoralis major and minor
- Oblique abdominal muscles
- Hamstrings
- Rectus femoris
- Tensor fasciae latae (TFL)
- Iliopsoas
- Short hip adductors
- Triceps surae
- Flexors of the upper extremity

Muscles with a Tendency to Weaken

- Deltoid
- Lower section of the trapezius
- Serratus anterior
- Gluteal muscles
- Rectus abdominis
- Deep neck benders
- Muscles at the floor of the mouth
- Vastus muscles
- Anterior tibial
- Toe extensors
- Peroneus muscles
- Extensors of the upper extremity

The function of muscle fibers, whether postural or phasic, appears not to be genetically conditioned but depends on the activity that the muscle has to execute. Chris Norris (in [41]), a British physiotherapist, writes that appropriate training conditions the amount of phasic or postural muscle fibers. Lin et al. (in [41]) were able to demonstrate that the postural or phasic property of a muscle depends on its innervation (or on the impulses that it receives). They verified this by transplanting the nerves of a phasic muscle into a postural muscle. Most likely, this also explains why we find different muscle properties in the case of malpositions (such as due to leg length differences) or ex-

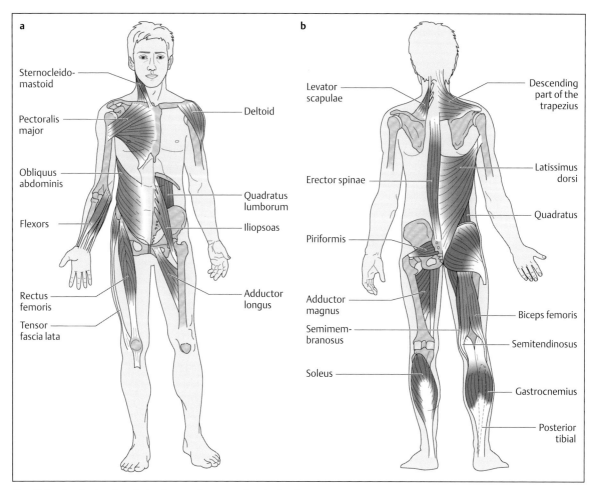

Fig. 6.1a, b   Postural and phasic muscles according to Janda.

cessive strain of certain muscle groups (such as in monotonous motion patterns during work).

For some muscles, classification into postural or phasic muscles is questionable. This applies to the scalene muscles, the oblique abdominal muscles, the gluteus muscles, and the deep neck muscles, as well as the peroneus muscles.

It is also remarkable that postural muscles are also found in the concavities of the spine and the extremities. Thus, from cranial to caudal:

- Neck stretchers
- Pectoralis major and minor
- Lumbar erector spinae
- Iliopsoas for the hip
- Hamstrings for the knee
- Peroneus muscle for the foot
- Flexors of the upper extremity

Janda's explanation for the formation of motion patterns is conditioned by evolution. It refers primarily to muscles with a stabilizing function in the gait.

For Waddell (in [41]), postural muscles are those with a stabilizing function, that is, static muscles. These are muscles that are able to tense continuously. Phasic muscles, on the other hand, are dynamic, responsible for movements. Postural and phasic muscles are antagonists in Waddell's view (see above).

6.4   Crossed Syndrome

The shoulder girdle and pelvic girdle commonly have very specific postural patterns:

▪ The Upper Crossed Syndrome

- Occiput and C1–C2 in hyperextension
- Protracted chin
- Lower cervical spinal column (CSC) and upper thoracic spinal column (TSC) under tension
- Rotation and abduction of the shoulder blades
- The shoulder joint socket is oriented forward.
- Levator scapulae and descending part of the trapezius pull the shoulder up.

The following muscles are involved (**Fig. 6.2a**):

Hypertonic Muscles
- Pectoralis major and minor
- Descending part of the trapezius
- Levator scapulae
- SCM

Hypotonic Muscles
- Ascending part of the trapezius
- Serratus anterior
- Rhomboid muscles

This results in tensions in the CSC as well as shoulder and arm pain.

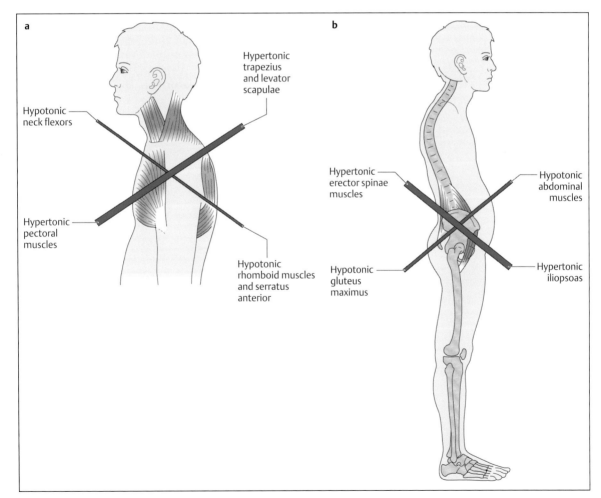

Fig. 6.2a, b   Upper and lower crossed syndrome according to Janda.

■ The Lower Crossed Syndrome

- Anteversion of the pelvis
- Hip flexion
- Lumbar spinal column (LSC) lordosis
- L5–S1 stress

The following muscles are involved (**Fig. 6.2b**):

Hypertonic Muscles

- Iliopsoas
- Rectus femoris
- TFL
- Adductors
- Erector spinae muscles of the LSC

Hypotonic Muscles

- Abdominal muscles
- Buttock muscles

Both syndromes together result in a kypholordotic spine.

Note: In principle, this "crossed syndrome" can be transferred to all other levels.

Example: Hypertonicity of the ischiocrural muscles and the foot extensors with hypotonicity of the quadriceps and triceps surae results in flexed position of the knee. Hypertonicity of the short adductors and quadratus lumborum with hypotonicity of the abductors and the biceps femoris result in a pelvic translation.

6.5   Practical Consequences

Some muscles tend toward hypertonicity and shortening; their functional antagonists, on the other hand, toward hypotonicity and weakening. This leads to malpositions. Analyzing posture offers clues for hypertonic and hypotonic muscles.

Before we can strengthen the hypotonic muscles, we have to detonify and stretch the hypertonic muscles with adequate treatment. We should focus more on muscle groups and motor patterns than on isolated muscles and their movements. Agonist and antagonist are dependent on the motion pattern.

Muscle properties (postural or phasic) can be influenced by adequate training. The amount of red or white fibers is dependent on function.

Stereotypes or motion patterns develop already in childhood. Traumas, psychological stress, and habits contribute to their formation. Long-lasting inactivity converts phasic muscle fibers into postural muscle fibers.

7 The Zink Patterns[40, 41, 81, 82]

J. Gordon Zink, American osteopath and longstanding docent in the department of osteopathy at Des Moines University, Iowa, devoted much of his life to studying the fasciae as well as the effects of fascial imbalances on posture and circulation. Thanks to Michael Kuchera (continuing education course, May 2004 in Berlin), who had the good fortune of working with Zink, the latter became known towards the end of his career as an osteopath with short treatments and fast results. He had developed a diagnostic method by which he was able to diagnose a dysfunctional region with just a few grips, as well as to determine just as quickly how effective his treatments had been.

Zink's research focused on posture, fascial tensions, and on their effects particularly on lymphatic circulation. Hence, he was able to determine that certain postural patterns were based on particular fascial tension patterns. He took advantage of this fact in both diagnosis and therapy.

For the purposes of his research, he examined **complaint-free people** as well as **people with complaints** and arrived at interesting conclusions: even in people who considered themselves completely healthy and indicated no complaints at all, Zink found a fascial torsion pattern. People without a fascial torsion pattern are extremely rare.

In all other "**asymmetrical**" people, Zink found a particular torsion pattern. He realized that the fascial pattern reverses at the functional junctions in the spine (occipitoatlantoaxial [OAA], cervicothoracic [CTJ], thoracolumbar [TLJ], and lumbosacral [LSJ]). In this context, fascial pattern refers to the ease with which a region permits rotation (ease bind). At the same time, it is an indication for fascial bias in the direction of the free movement.

In 80% of the complaint-free population, he found the following patterns:
- OAA: leftward torsion
- Upper thoracic aperture: rightward torsion
- Lower thoracic aperture: leftward torsion
- Pelvis: rightward torsion

Because this was the most common fascial pattern in healthy people, Zink called it the "common compensatory pattern" (CCP).

In the remaining 20% of the **complaint-free population**, he found the opposite pattern:
- OAA: rightward torsion
- Upper thoracic aperture: leftward torsion
- Lower thoracic aperture: rightward torsion
- Pelvis: leftward torsion

This pattern he called "uncommon compensatory pattern" (UCCP). When the fascial biases change at each of the anatomical transitions, this means that the person has found a homeostatic postural adaptation. The organism has been able to compensate successfully, even if it was unable to adopt the "ideal" adaptive pattern without torsions.

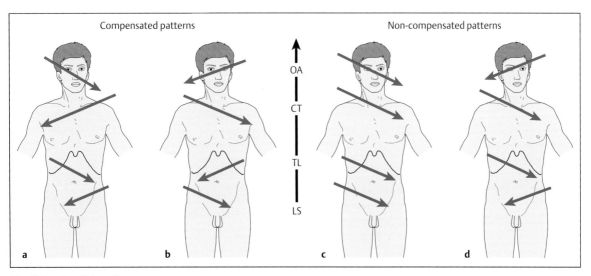

Fig. 7.1a–d Zink patterns.

In patients, that is, people with complaints, we find none of these three patterns. People who present neither with the ideal fascial pattern nor with one of the two compensatory torsion patterns (CCP or UCCP) (**Fig. 7.1a, b**) frequently have fascial preferences in the same direction in two or even several transitions. In this case, we speak of non-compensatory fascial patterns (NCP) (**Fig. 7.1c, d**). **Zink posited that the cause for this inability of the organism to adapt was found in micro- or macro-traumas that prevented the body from adapting to the law of gravity.**

Two facts stand out in this model:
- The reversal of fascial bias takes place in regions where we find diaphragms (anatomical or functional ones). As we know, these play an eminent role in venolymphatic circulation as active pumps.
- The areas of reversal are also those areas in which a lordosis converts to a kyphosis or vice versa. These are also areas of reversal in scoliotic curvatures.

Note: When we further pursue this notion of diaphragms and transitions, we cannot avoid discussing the sphenobasilar synchondrosis (SBS) and the cerebellar tentorium. We are all aware of the significance of the tentorium for the circulation of the head. From cranial osteopathy, we also know how important the SBS is for postural adjustments. If this has not become obvious from what we have written above, we hope that the following sections will make this evident.

The upper thoracic aperture or the cervicothoracic diaphragm is a functional diaphragm. The so-called anatomical thoracic inlet is formed by the articulation of the sternum, the first pair of ribs, and the first thoracic vertebra. The functional thoracic inlet is identical to the clinical thoracic inlet and is formed by the manubrium, the angle of Louis, the first pair of ribs laterally, and the first four thoracic vertebrae. In this thoracic aperture, we find the two pulmonal apexes, as well as vessels, nerves, trachea, and esophagus, which constitute the upper mediastinum. These structures are enveloped by Sibson's fascia, which originates from the fascia of the two longus colli muscles (reaching down to T4–T5) and the visceral leaf of the scalene cover. It covers the apexes of the lung and attaches to the vessel trunks of the thoracic inlet, to grow together with the pleural dome. This Sibson's fascia is the real cervicothoracic diaphragm.

7.1   The Composition of the Zink Patterns

As part of our effort to compare the various models of thought with each other and to find analogies, we will now describe the muscle groups responsible for the torsion patterns, and the involved segments (**Fig. 7.2**).

■ Occiput-Atlas-Axis

Vertebrae

- Occiput
- Atlas
- Axis

Responsible Muscles

- Rectus capitis superior, inferior, lateralis, and anterior
- Obliquus minor, major
- Sternocleidomastoideus (SCM) and superior part of the trapezius

We consider the SCM muscle under all circumstances as part of those muscles that play a role for the head joints, since its main function concerns the head. The trapezius is certainly involved in both regions, the occiput-atlas-axis (OAA) and the thoracic aperture.

Segments

- Cervical plexus

Some Osteopathic Considerations

- The atlas is the socket for the head. All cranial problems affect the OAA complex and vice versa.
- The OAA is a key area of the cranial parasympathicus.
- The suboccipital musculature in general and the SCM because of its attachment to the suture are able to irritate the occipitomastoid (OM) suture.
- Hypertonicity can affect the jugular foramen. In addition, the nodose (inferior) ganglion of the vagus nerve lies covered by fasciae between the lateral mass of the atlas and the jugular foramen.
- Besides the lumbosacral junction and the lower ankle joint, the OAA is the most important adaptation zone for posture.
- The suboccipital muscles are richly supplied with muscle spindles and therefore extremely important for posture.

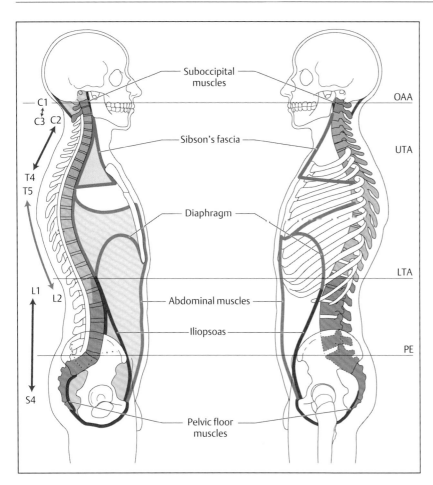

Fig. 7.2 Myofascial components and vertebral segments of the Zink patterns.

Upper Thoracic Aperture

Vertebrae

- C3–T4 (T5)

Muscles

- Long neck muscles
- The upper three to four intercostal muscles
- Scalene muscles
- Longus colli
- Scapular muscles

Segments

- Brachial plexus
- Thoracic segments T1–T5

Some Osteopathic Considerations

- The upper thoracic aperture (UTA) is the gateway to venolymphatic circulation. The cervical fasciae wrap all vessels in the UTA.
- The stellate ganglion lies in front of the head of the first rib.
- The sympathetic nerve supply of all head and thoracic organs comes from the segments T1–T5.
- A functional relationship exists between the upper thoracic spinal column (TSC) and the cervical spinal column (CSC).
- The CTJ is the junction from a less mobile to a mobile zone.
- Interrelation between the upper extremity and the CTJ.

Lower Thoracic Aperture

Vertebrae

- T6–L3

Muscles

- Diaphragm muscles
- Abdominal muscles
- The last seven intercostal muscles

Segments

- T6–T9: major splanchnic nerve
- T9–T12: minor splanchnic nerve
- Pelvic splanchnic nerve

Some Osteopathic Considerations

- Significance of the diaphragm for thoracic respiration, circulation, organ function, and posture.
- Functional unity between diaphragm, quadratus lumborum, and iliopsoas.
- Sympathetic nerve supply of all abdominal organs.
- Connection to the CSC via the phrenic nerve, which arises from the segments C3, C4, and C5.
- The diaphragm plays a central role for pressure conditions in the abdomen and thorax and therefore for all body functions.
  Example: An increase of abdominal pressure moves the diaphragm upward to keep the pressure gradient constant between the thoracic and abdominal cavities. This increases pressure in the thorax, which eventually stresses respiration and circulation. With greater physical exertion, the auxiliary musculature of respiration must be increasingly activated. Both facts, the changed pressure conditions as well as the strain on the auxiliary musculature of respiration, affect the posture of the spine. When the diaphragm functions at a high level for a long time, this changes not only the axes of movement in the organs, but also the orientation of the respiratory movements in the diaphragm. This in turn affects the entire mobilization of the organs that depends on respiration.
- The iliopsoas and quadratus lumborum are significant muscles for the posture of the pelvis and lumbar spinal column (LSC). Their nerve supply comes from the upper LSC.
- The TLJ is a key area for torsions of the spinal column.

Pelvis

Vertebrae

- L4, L5
- Iliosacral joints

Muscles

- Iliopsoas
- Gluteus muscles
- Pelvic floor muscles

Segments

- L4–S4
- Lumbosacral plexus
- Sacral parasympathetic nerve

Some Osteopathic Considerations

- Like OAA and ankle joints, the LSJ is a hinge for posture.
- Functionally, L4 and L5 belong to the pelvis. Their action is connected to that of the ilium and sacrum via the iliolumbar ligaments.
- The stability of the LSJ depends on the integrity of all the pelvic joints.
- The iliosacral joints are very susceptible to traumatic dysfunctions. A badly suspended landing on one or both legs after a jump or a fall on the back or buttocks (infants) are often the beginning of creeping malpositions and dysfunctions.
- Leg length differences sooner or later lead to pelvic torsion (± 70% of the population have legs of different lengths!).
- The craniosacral connection has been discussed in another chapter (see pp. 45ff). In this context, we just want to add that Chapman (Chapman reflexes) considered the pelvis a key area in cases of endocrine disorders.
- Connections to the organs consist of fascial attachments on the one hand, and the sacral parasympathetic nerve via neural connections on the other hand.

7.2 Practical Application of the Zink Patterns

The Zink patterns can be applied in diagnosis as well as in therapy. Every junction (OAA, CTJ, diaphragm, pelvis) carries a particular significance for a certain region:

■ Occiput-Atlas-Axis

• Head: Dominant cranial problems lead to suboccipital tensions and dysfunctions.
Example: Problems of the temporomandibular joints, sinuses, eyes, and so on.
Note: We purposely do not use the terms "primary lesion" or "primary dysfunction" because we believe that every person in the course of childhood acquires a certain pattern that makes them susceptible to certain dysfunctions. This notion is also found in typology (Vannier) and homeopathy.

■ Upper Thoracic Aperture (Fig. 7.3)

• Lower CSC
• Upper extremities
• Upper TSC and ribs
• Thoracic and cervical organs
Note: It goes without saying that a dominant problem of a thoracic organ also irritates the diaphragm and thereby the corresponding segments. With a few exceptions, however, the test for the UTA gives more obvious results.

■ Lower Thoracic Aperture

• Vertebral segments T6–L3
• The last six ribs
• Upper abdominal organs
• CSC—segments C3–C5 (phrenic nerve)
Note: The same applies here as for the UTA. Because of its functional significance for the entire organism, the diaphragm is frequently affected. The rotation test allows us to compare torsion patterns at the various junctions. A dominant test at the lower thoracic aperture (LTA) strongly suggests that the above-mentioned structures play a key role in this pathological process.

■ Pelvis

• Vertebrae T12–L5
• Iliosacral joint (ISJ), symphysis
• Lower extremities
• Lower abdominal organs
Note: The quadratus lumborum and iliopsoas muscles constitute a connection between the TLJ and the pelvis. Both of these regions influence each other as well the upper TSC and the OAA region.

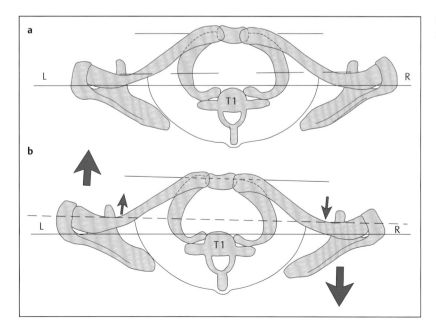

Fig. 7.3a, b Torsion of the upper thoracic aperture.

Knowing the significance of the diaphragm for circulation, it is worthwhile treating it in case of tensions, to influence pressure conditions in the cavities and to improve venolymphatic circulation. For a long-lasting effect, it is necessary to treat the structure(s) in the related areas that prevent(s) smooth functioning of the diaphragm. Often, manipulating a vertebra or treating an organ complex suffices.

In addition to examining torsion patterns, Zink developed his own diagnostic procedure to control the efficacy of the treatment. Having treated the affected region of the body, he exerted pressure with one hand on the abdomen of the standing patient. The patient now was supposed to tell the therapist spontaneously whether they felt a heat sensation spreading from the cervical region downward along the spinal column and where this heat sensation stopped. The place where the heat stopped marked the region that was treated next.

This test is based on the effect that an increase in intra-abdominal pressure causes a build-up of venous blood towards the azygos system and the venous plexi in the spinal column. This creates a slight heat flush in the area with increased circulation. The higher muscle tension and the blockage in the spinal column slow down circulation and thereby the heating of the tissue.

For us, the Zink patterns are an interesting diagnostic tool. They allow us to find the affected spinal column segment and give additional information on the dominant muscle chain.

Example: In a rightward rotation of the upper thoracic aperture, the left shoulder is positioned anterior and the right shoulder posterior. If the left shoulder is comparatively harder to press backward than the right one is to press forward, a left anterior chain dominates.

8 Myofascial Chains—A Model

As already mentioned in the introduction, we consider muscles, as the organ of myofascial chains, to play an important role in all bodily functions. Also, while their main function centers on locomotion and maintaining equilibrium, we should not disregard their contribution to other vital functions. Thus, they are important for respiration, digestion, and circulation. Their significance becomes obvious in the case of dysfunctions, and when Still states that the fasciae are where we must look for the source of diseases and also where we should initiate treatment, this only emphasizes their significance.[140]

The myofascial tissue belongs to the connective tissue and contains the subcutaneous and deep fasciae, as well as the skin, muscles, tendons, and ligaments. Schultz and Feitis refer to the fascial system as an endless network that connects everything with everything.[132]

The fascial connections are arranged not coincidentally or anarchically, but functionally. The spinal column plays a special role here. It serves as anchor for practically all fascial connections, similar to a ship's mast to which the ropes are tied. The ropes stabilize the mast, but the mast holds the sails. As long as the ropes are taut and the mast is anchored solidly, the sails function. Our trunk consists of a number of fascial planes that are connected to the spinal column and balance each other out.

We can distinguish between three ventral and three dorsal (muscle) fascial planes on the trunk:

- An outer plane with the latissimus dorsi and trapezius in the back and the pectoralis muscles and serratus anterior in front. These are muscles whose main task consists of mobilizing the arms.
- The middle layer consists of the paravertebral muscles and both serratus posterior muscles in the back, and the longus colli, intercostal muscles, abdominal muscles, and psoas ventrally. These muscles directly affect the spinal column (even though the intercostal and abdominal muscles use the ribs as levers).
- The deep layer consists of fascial structures: dorsally the nuchal ligament and ligamentous apparatus of the vertebral arches, and ventrally the central tendon with the serosae of the organs.

The three ventral and three dorsal myofascial layers are able to balance out the spinal column (the mast). In the case of hypertonicity on one side, the other side gives a little. As a result, the mast stands a little askew, but is still stable. This reflects the interplay of agonist and antagonist. The same model can be applied in the frontal plane. The myofascial structures of one side must adjust to the tensions on the other side to stabilize the spinal column.

We are convinced that when the equilibrium is concerned, especially when a position has to be maintained for a longer time, the organism utilizes all available means as economically as possible and thereby affects the other bodily functions as little as possible. Thoracic respiration and cellular respiration, as well as venolymphatic circulation must all continue to function.

The curvature of the spinal column contributes to its stability. We can therefore assume that the vertebrae act in such a way that they position the spinal column under strain to enable the physiological curves to counteract any pressure. In asymmetrical strain (such as weight in one hand), this results in scoliotic posture.

The individual spinal column segments herein move around Littlejohn's pivotal vertebrae (see Chapter 5, pp. 62ff). The pivotal vertebrae can sometimes be a segment higher or lower. As a rule, however, they are C2, C5, T4, T9, L3, and L5/S1.

The muscles need solid support to be able to execute their tasks optimally. This is provided by other muscles. This leads to the formation of muscle chains. When standing, the feet are the fixed point for the muscle chains. They are therefore of particular significance in posture.

A further factor that contributes to stability but also facilitates harmonious movements in all planes is the arrangement of muscles in the shape of **lemniscates**. According to Wahrig, a lemniscate is "an arrangement in the shape of a figure eight on its side." In fact, all muscles with the exception of the rectus abdominis run along a more or less diagonal or swinging course. The muscles follow in chains in such a way that they form loops that pass harmoniously from one plane to the other (**Fig. 8.1**).

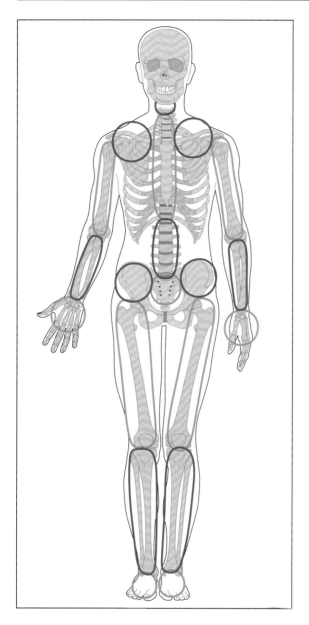

Fig 8.1   Motor units.

Littlejohn's pivots and the joints in the extremities are located more or less exactly on the crossings of lemniscates or in the center of loops. Here we can see that Littlejohn's model is not only structural but also functional.

The arrangement of the muscles in lemniscates facilitates a very energy-efficient execution of smooth movements in all planes. It becomes possible to convert potential energy into kinetic energy. Thereby, the effect of a spiral or spring is obtained (see the gait study in Chapter 3, p. 39). An additional advantage is the fact that pressure on the vessels, thorax, and abdomen is reduced.

Note: The greater the load that we must transport, the greater our muscular exertion becomes because we can no longer utilize the momentum of the movement. At the same time, this increases the strain on the joints, respiration, and circulation. Muscle contractions and joint blockages have the same effect.

8.1   Muscle Chains

In the preceding chapters, we have introduced a number of muscle chain models. While some have certain similarities (Busquet and Chauffour, both from the French school), others are very specialized (Myers, Struyf-Denis). Each of the authors described their model from a particular perspective. For Rolfers, for example, certain aspects dominate more than for osteopaths or physiotherapists.

In addition, we described the mechanical aspect of cranial osteopathy, the Zink patterns, and Littlejohn's model of the spinal column. Furthermore, we determined that one of the main functions of the locomotor system, namely the gait, reproduces the behavior of the spinal column and the pelvis, as described by Sutherland, Zink, and Littlejohn in their models.

For us, it is obvious that it is the muscles that form these patterns. This is by no means in contradiction to Sutherland's craniosacral theory. No matter whether a pattern is triggered by the skull, the trunk, or the extremities, the rest of the body adopts the same pattern (for economical reasons; to avoid burdening the brain). This is important from a craniosacral perspective because it allows the primary respiratory mechanism (PRM) to function free of stress.

This also explains why the segment or the skull is adjusted in the lesion pattern during treatments with the Sutherland techniques. This allows for a flexion and extension of the PRM that is as free as possible.

The muscle chain model that we propose differs from the other models in two essential respects:

1. We are convinced that flexion and extension alternate in the spinal column and upper extremity as they do in the lower extremity. The definition of flexion is the bringing together of both ends of an arch; extension is the distancing of the ends of an arch. The spinal column consists of three arches, of which two are dorsally concave, and one is ventrally concave. Accordingly, flexion of the cervical spinal column (CSC) is a posterior flexion, that of the thoracic spinal column (TSC) is an anterior flexion, and that of the lumbar spinal column (LSC) is again a posterior flexion.

   This perspective on flexion and extension of the spinal column is interesting in that it accords with Sutherland's model. Cranial flexion corresponds to an extension of the spinal column, that is, an extension of the three arches. Cranial extension is the opposite.

   On the upper extremity, we also find an alternation between flexion and extension (upper arm in extension, elbow flexed, fist extended, and fingers flexed, see the position of the arm during writing). We believe that a slight flexion in the elbow and a medium position between pro- and supination constitutes the neutral position of the lower arm.

2. In our opinion, there are only two muscle chains in each half of the body:
   - a flexion chain; and
   - an extension chain.

As described by Sutherland, external rotation and abduction are associated with flexion, and internal rotation and adduction with extension (see **Figs. 8.2** and **8.3**). This results in the following combinations:

- Flexion + abduction + external rotation
- Extension + adduction + internal rotation

Note: We point out again that cranial flexion corresponds to extension in the parietal plane.

The arrangement of muscles in the shape of lemniscates permits a continuity of myofascial chains between individual spinal column segments and thereby creates connections between right and left. The same is true for the extremities.

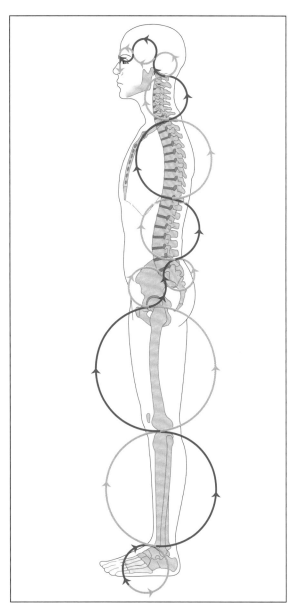

Fig. 8.2 Behavior of individual motor units in case of dominance of a flexion pattern (*bright blue*) or extension pattern (*dark blue*).

The inhibition of the antagonist and the crossed stretch reflex are the neurophysiological foundations for the formation of torsion patterns.

Before describing the muscle chains, we first want to describe the functional motor units of the skeleton:

Cranium

- Sphenoid with facial and frontal bones
- Occiput with temporal bones, parietal bones, and mandible.

Spinal Column

- Atlas + axis
- C3–T4
- T4–T12
- T12–L5
- Sacrum

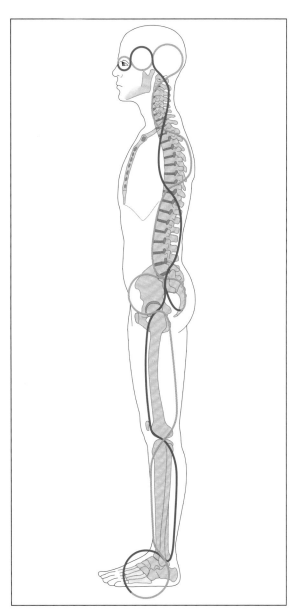

Fig. 8.3 Flexion chain (*dark blue*) and extension chain (*bright blue*).

Pelvic Girdle and Lower Limb

- Ilium
- Thigh
- Lower leg
- Upper ankle joint
- Lower ankle joint and foot

Shoulder Girdle and Upper Limb

- Shoulder blade
- Upper arm
- Lower arm
- Wrist joint
- Finger

The individual units function together like cogwheels.

Before we populate the muscle chains with muscles (see **Figs. 8.4** and **8.5**), we need to stress once more that the brain does not recognize individual muscles, but only functions. These movements are executed by muscle groups (agonists and synergists).

In movements that involve more than one plane, the involved muscles can change. It is also possible that only a part of a muscle is involved. This is made possible by the polysegmental innervation of muscles. In the extremities, and particularly in the distal areas of the arm and leg, it becomes difficult to assign individual muscles specifically. If therapists cannot obtain a clear picture by visual inspection, they sometimes have to palpate the individual compartments and compare.

In the clinical section of this book, we will see that we can find the dominant muscle chain by means of simple tests.

■ Flexion Chain

A dominance of the flexion chain coincides with a cranial mechanism in extension (internal rotation).

Cranium

- Occiput posterior
- Sphenobasilar synchondrosis (SBS) low
- Sphenoid: body low
- Greater wings posterior and medial
- Peripheral bones in internal rotation

Spinal Column

- **Occipitoatlantoaxial (OAA)**: occiput in flexion, atlas anterior in relation.
  Responsible muscles: rectus capitis anterior/longus capitis.

Note: The central tendon is also able to pull the SBS into extension. It is not a muscle, but the weight of the organs can exert a pull caudally. This is the case in this pattern because the thorax is in exhalation position and therefore cannot assist in lifting the organs.

- **C3–T4**: In extension, the lordosis is increased globally.
Responsible muscles: low paravertebral musculature between C3 and T4, semispinalis capitis, longissimus capitis, splenius capitis, splenius cervicis.
- **T4–T12**: The thoracic vertebrae are in flexion and the ribs in exhalatory position.
Responsible muscles: intercostal and abdominal muscles.
Note: It may surprise some readers that we consider the abdominal muscles as thoracic muscles. Embryologically, they belong to the thoracic segments from which they are also innervated (T5–L1). By their connection with the last seven ribs, they pull the thorax into flexion.
- **T12–L5**: The lumbar spinal column is extended.
Responsible muscles: lumbar paravertebral muscles, quadratus lumborum.
Note: The continuity of the chain is preserved by the quadratus lumborum muscle, which is connected to the 12th rib and with the abdominal fascia.
- **Sacrum**: The sacrum makes a nutation. The basis moves forward and downward and the coccyx moves backward and downward.
Responsible muscles: multifidi muscles in the lumbosacral area.
Note: The thoracolumbar fascia is also involved in this process. Its lower leaf serves as the base for the multifidi muscles and the quadratus lumborum.

Pelvic Girdle and Lower Limb

- **Ilium**: The ilium makes a dorsal rotation under the simultaneous pull of the abdominal and gluteal muscles.
Responsible muscles: abdominal muscles, gluteal muscles, TFL.
- **Hip**: The hip is extended.
Responsible muscles: gluteal muscles.
Note: We have a continuous chain between the abdominal and gluteal muscles via the iliac crest on the one hand, and the quadratus lumborum and gluteal muscles via the thoracolumbar fascia on the other. For the gluteal muscles to turn the ilium dorsally, they must be firmly supported at the femur.

This is provided by two mechanisms:
- The gluteus maximus is connected to the tensor fasciae latae (TFL) via the iliotibial tract. The TFL prevents an external rotation of the hip, which allows the gluteus maximus to exert a pull on the ilium. The lower layer of the gluteus maximus is connected to the vastus externus, which is activated by the same motion pattern. A pull of the vastus externus in addition stabilizes the gluteus maximus.
- A rotation of the ilium backward raises the ramus of the pubis. The adductors are hereby stretched. They will reclaim the lost length on the other end, namely the femur. In a backward rotation of the ilium, the adductors pull the leg into adduction and internal rotation. This results in two positions for the lower extremity: **extension + adduction + internal rotation**.
- **Knee**: The knee is stretched.
Responsible muscles: quadriceps.
- **Upper ankle joint**: The upper ankle joint is in plantar flexion, the talus is pressed forward between the mortise and calcaneus.
Responsible muscles: triceps surae and flexors.
- **Lower ankle joint and foot**: Dominance of the flexion chain results in eversion of the foot with a drop in the arch. The talus plays the main role herein. Free of muscle attachments, it is pressed forward medially by pressure from the mortise. This shifts the weight to the inner edge of the foot. The cuboid bone makes an external rotation and the navicular bone an internal rotation.
Responsible muscles: extensor digitorum longus, tibialis anterior, extensor hallucis longus, extensor digitorum longus.

Shoulder Girdle and Upper Limb

- **Shoulder blade**: The shoulder blade stands in abduction; the glenoid cavity is oriented forward and outward. This presents as rolled-in shoulders (Janda's upper crossed syndrome).
Responsible muscles: descending part of the trapezius, pectoralis minor.
Depending on which muscle pull dominates, the shoulder is depressed or raised.
- **Upper arm**: The arm is in adduction–internal rotation and extension. The pectoralis major is pulled because the thorax is in exhalatory position. It regains the lost length by moving the arm into adduction–internal rotation. The anterior shoulder exerts tension on the latissimus dorsi, which tries to regain its normal length by extending the shoulder.
Responsible muscles: pectoralis major, latissimus dorsi, teres major, subscapularis.

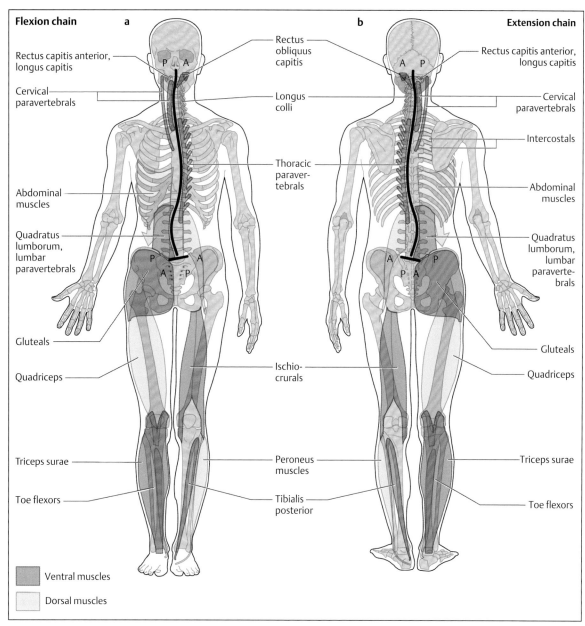

Flexion chain   a

- Rectus capitis anterior, longus capitis
- Cervical paravertebrals
- Abdominal muscles
- Quadratus lumborum, lumbar paravertebrals
- Gluteals
- Quadriceps
- Triceps surae
- Toe flexors

b   **Extension chain**

- Rectus capitis anterior, longus capitis
- Cervical paravertebrals
- Intercostals
- Abdominal muscles
- Quadratus lumborum, lumbar paravertebrals
- Gluteals
- Quadriceps
- Triceps surae
- Toe flexors

(center labels)
- Rectus obliquus capitis
- Longus colli
- Thoracic paravertebrals
- Ischio-crurals
- Peroneus muscles
- Tibialis posterior

◼ Ventral muscles
◻ Dorsal muscles

Fig. 8.4a, b   **a** Ventral view:
– Flexion chain: right half of the body
– Extension chain: left half of the body.

b Dorsal view:
– Flexion chain: right half of the body
– Extension chain: left half of the body.

- **Lower arm**: The elbow is flexed and the lower arm in pronation.
  Responsible muscles: biceps brachii, brachialis, pronators.
- **Hand**: The wrist is in extension.
  Responsible muscles: hand extensors.
- **Fingers**: The fingers are flexed.
  Responsible muscles: finger flexors.

Here we find the reversal of flexion and extension, as well as the dominance of the extension–adduction–internal rotation aspect. Contrary to the lower extremity, where we find a global extension, however, we see a flexion here. We explain this as a remnant of archaic reflexes, as we know them from spastic hemiplegics.

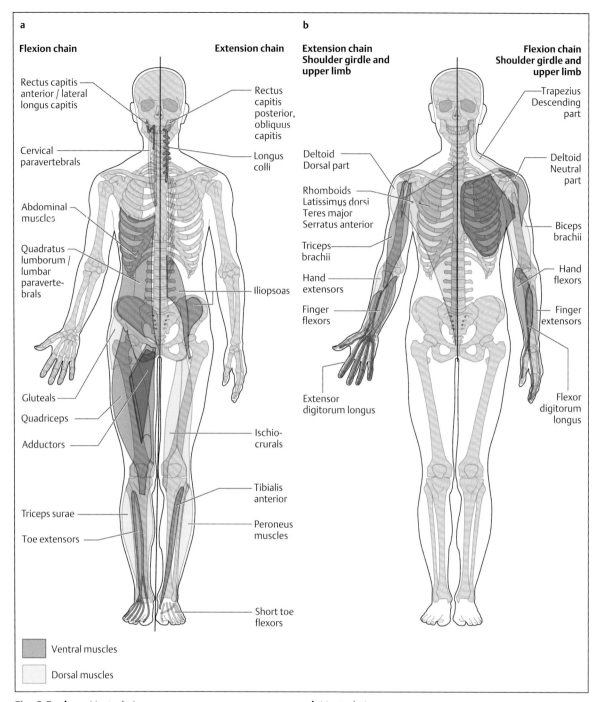

a

Flexion chain

Rectus capitis anterior / lateral longus capitis

Cervical paravertebrals

Abdominal muscles

Quadratus lumborum / lumbar paraverte- brals

Gluteals

Quadriceps

Adductors

Triceps surae

Toe extensors

Extension chain

Rectus capitis posterior, obliquus capitis

Longus colli

Iliopsoas

Ischio- crurals

Tibialis anterior

Peroneus muscles

Short toe flexors

b

Extension chain Shoulder girdle and upper limb

Deltoid Dorsal part

Rhomboids Latissimus dorsi Teres major Serratus anterior

Triceps brachii

Hand extensors

Finger flexors

Extensor digitorum longus

Flexion chain Shoulder girdle and upper limb

Trapezius Descending part

Deltoid Neutral part

Biceps brachii

Hand flexors

Finger extensors

Flexor digitorum longus

▨ Ventral muscles

☐ Dorsal muscles

Fig. 8.5a, b   **a** Ventral view:
– Flexion chain left
– Extension chain right.

b Ventral view:
– Extension chain of the shoulder girdle and upper limb left
– Flexion chain of the shoulder girdle and upper limb right.

Fig. 8.5c ▶

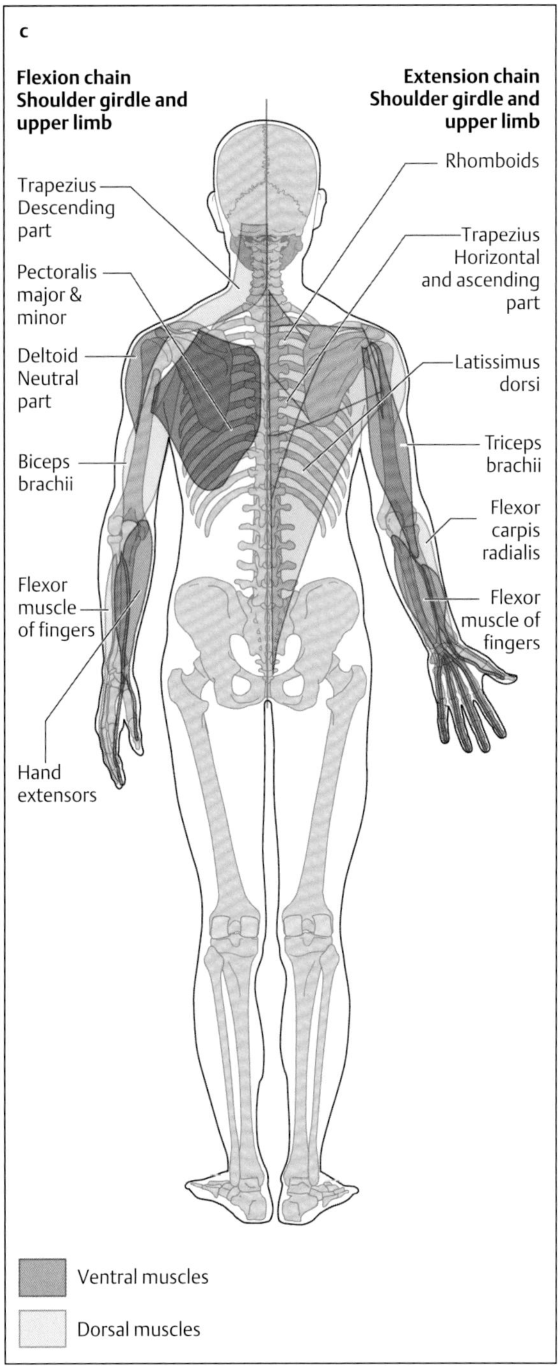

c

Flexion chain
Shoulder girdle and
upper limb

Trapezius
Descending
part

Pectoralis
major &
minor

Deltoid
Neutral
part

Biceps
brachii

Flexor
muscle
of fingers

Hand
extensors

Extension chain
Shoulder girdle and
upper limb

Rhomboids

Trapezius
Horizontal
and ascending
part

Latissimus
dorsi

Triceps
brachii

Flexor
carpis
radialis

Flexor
muscle of
fingers

Ventral muscles

Dorsal muscles

Fig. 8.5c Dorsal view:
– Extension chain of the shoulder girdle and upper limb right
– Flexion chain of the shoulder girdle and upper limb left.

Extension Chain

We find an extension chain in combination with a cranial flexion pattern.

Cranium

- Occiput anterior
- SBS high
- Sphenoid: body high
- Greater wings: anterior and lateral
- Peripheral skull bones in external rotation

Spinal Column

- **OAA**: Occiput in extension, atlas relatively posterior. Responsible muscles: major and minor rectus capitis posterior, superior and inferior obliquus capitis, sternocleidomastoideus (SCM).
  Note: The descending part of the trapezius is able to move the occiput into the extension. Its main function focuses, however, on the shoulder.
- **C3–T4**: The cervical spinal column is straightened. Responsible muscle: longus colli.
- **T4–T12**: The thoracic spinal column is straightened. Responsible muscles: thoracic paravertebral muscles, superior and inferior serratus posterior, and thoracic fascia.
  Note: Straightening the thoracic spinal column brings the thorax into inhalatory position. This is made possible by the reciprocal inhibition of the abdominal muscles. The diaphragm is thereby brought up higher, which moves it into a better working position.
- **T12–L5**: The lordosis of the lumbar spinal column is removed. Responsible muscles: iliopsoas (see p. 91).
- **Sacrum**: The sacrum makes a contranutation. The base moves backward and the coccyx forward. Responsible muscles: pelvic floor muscles.
  Note: The pelvic floor is lifted and therefore more operative.

Pelvic Girdle and Lower Limb

- **Ilium**: The ISJ makes an anterior rotation of the ilium. Responsible muscles: iliopsoas, sartorius, rectus femoris, adductors.
- **Hip**: The hip is bent. Responsible muscles: rectus femoris, sartorius, adductors (besides adductor magnus), iliopsoas.
  Note: The forward rotation of the ilium and flexion of the hip cause the gluteus maximus to stretch. It compensates by increased abduction and external rotation. The piriformis assists the sacrum in the dorsal

turn, but at the same time rotates the thigh outward. This results in a flexion with external rotation and abduction in the leg, which fits the cranial flexion model as described by Sutherland.

- **Knee**: The knee is bent.
Responsible muscles: hamstrings.
The anterior rotation of the ilium shifts the tuberosity of the ischium dorsally, as a result of which the *ischiocrural musculature* is tensed. This can be reduced by flexion of the knee.
Note: In stance, the knee flexion is often inconspicuous; the knee is even frequently in recurvatum. This is the result of a relative release of tension in the sacrotuberal ligaments due to the opposite rotation of the ilium and sacrum. Consequently, the entire pelvis has a tendency to anteversion. The body balances this by shifting the buttocks backward. Such patients present with a "false hyperlordosis." The lower lumbar spinal column is in flexion and the lower thoracic spinal column compensates for this with a lordosis. Typical examples are pregnant women and pot-bellied men.
- **Upper ankle joint**: The foot is in dorsal extension. The talus is pressed backward between the mortise and calcaneus.
Responsible muscles: tibialis anterior, dorsal extensors of the toes.
- **Lower ankle joint and foot**: The foot makes an inversion. The muscles of the sole of the foot increase the arch of the foot. The toes are bent. Depending on which flexors dominate, the result is hammer or claw toes.
Responsible muscles: flexors, peroneus muscles, tibialis posterior.

Shoulder Girdle and Upper Limb

- **Shoulder blade**: The shoulder blade is in adduction and lies on top of the ribs. The shoulder is pulled back and the glenoid cavity is oriented laterally.
Responsible muscles: trapezius, rhomboid muscles, serratus anterior.
Note: The inhalatory position of the chest and straightened thoracic spinal column contribute to this presentation.
- **Upper arm**: The arm is in flexion or rather, less in extension than in the flexion pattern.
Responsible muscles: clavicular part of the pectoralis major, deltoid, coracobrachialis.
Note: When the shoulder is stabilized backward by the shoulder blade fixators, the pectoralis minor and major muscles assist the ribs in their upward pull. The latissimus dorsi becomes relatively relaxed due to the posteriorization of the shoulder, as a result of which the pectoralis major is able to pull the arm forward together with the anterior aspect of the deltoid and coracobrachialis. The lateral orientation of the glenoid cavity brings the arm into an external rotation. When the deltoid adds some abduction, this causes the following position: **flexion–abduction–external rotation**.
- **Lower arm**: The elbow is stretched and the lower arm supinated.
Responsible muscles: triceps brachii, supinator, brachioradialis.
- **Hand**: The wrist is bent (or rather, less stretched).
Responsible muscles: hand and finger flexors.
- **Fingers**: The fingers are stretched.
Responsible muscles: finger extensors.

8.2 Summary and Conclusions of the Flexion and Extension Chains

■ Flexion Chain

This pattern can dominate bilaterally or unilaterally. In a bilateral pattern, it results in kypholordotic posture with extended legs and tendency to flat feet. The shoulders are pulled forward; the arms are bent and rotated inward. The thorax is sunken and the abdomen more or less vaulted forward, in spite of a taught abdominal wall.

On the cranial level, this is an extension pattern according to Sutherland, with the SBS in extension and peripheral bones rotated inward. The sinuses are narrower. The cerebellar tentorium is more oblique. The head is smaller and the face more elongated.

The low position of the thorax lowers the diaphragm. This causes a pull on the central tendon, which further emphasizes the cranial extension position. The low position of the thorax provides less support to the abdominal organs, which favors sagging.

It is notable that this position matches the asthenic, passive type. Some authors also refer to the extension stage of the craniosacral mechanism as a passive stage. This concerns the return from the active flexion stage. The flexion position corresponds to the "relaxed position." It is the position that gravity forces on the organism.

The spinal column curvature is increased, which causes tensions in the ligaments. The nutation of the sacrum and the dorsal rotation of the iliac bones tighten the ligaments of the lumbosacral junction (LSJ). The dorsal rotation of the pelvis and the extension of the hip tighten the ventral ligaments of the hip joint.

The knee extension locks the knee through the cruciate ligaments. Only the foot is "unlocked" and becomes the weak point with the diaphragms. The physiological self-locking mechanism of the spinal column and lower extremities demands less muscle activity for stabilization. This could explain the weak muscle tone and asthenic type.

▪ Extension Chain

This pattern can occur unilaterally or bilaterally. In the extension pattern (cranial flexion), the spinal column is extended and the extremities bent. The organism is ready for action or engaged in action. Cranial flexion is the active stage of the craniosacral rhythm PRM.

The SBS is in flexion (high) and the peripheral skull bones are in external rotation. The foramina of the skull are open and the venous sinuses wide. Everything is prepared for a good circulation.

The cerebellar tentorium stands high, similar to the thoracic and pelvic diaphragms. Even the plantar aponeurosis is arched, ready for the propulsion stage of the gait.

The inhalatory position of the chest and the high position of the diaphragm support the abdominal organs and protect the lower abdomen from excessive pressure. The high diaphragm reduces the pull on the central tendon, which allows the SBS to move in flexion.

8.3   Torsion

A torsion pattern forms when one side of the body develops a dominant chain. The "crossed extension reflex" then leads to the formation of a torsion pattern. The result is scoliotic posture. If this occurs in early childhood, a large c-shaped curve forms because the lordoses are not yet fully developed. The diagonal course of the muscle fibers as well as the continuity of the fascial planes between the two halves of the body facilitate torsion. This is particularly obvious at the trunk, where we have, for example, an identical course of the fibers at the back in the latissimus dorsi and the gluteus maximus, and ventrally in the pectoralis major and external oblique muscle.

This arrangement of the fibers originated out of a functional need. During gait, the pelvic and shoulder girdles—as already explained—move in opposite directions. This causes the torsion of the trunk. Structure has adapted to function. The diagonal chains can be followed into the extremities at will. For example, we can follow the dorsal chain in the latissimus and gluteus maximus caudally through the vastus externus, which extends via the patellar retinaculum to the medial side of the knee. Here we have a dorsal chain that moves into a ventral one.

A similar ventral chain can be described as follows. If we start, for example, with the left pectoralis major, we arrive, via the right external oblique muscle, at the right ilium. The right adductors create continuity to the right leg. The short head of the biceps femoris extends the central part of the adductor magnus up to the head of the fibula. The ventral extension of the adductor magnus is the vastus medialis, which creates a connection to the other side of the leg, similar to the

vastus lateralis. From here on, we can follow the chain on through the tibialis anterior or the peroneus muscles.

The connections between the individual muscles and the continuous transitions from one side to the other and from the back to the front result in a network of loops, comparable to lemniscates.

Scoliosis, as well as scoliotic posture, is a holistic process that occurs in the three planes of the body. The anteroposterior curves of the skeleton are maintained. It is as if the entire trunk had turned around a vertical axis, while the feet had stayed in place. The mechanics of the spinal column and the sensitivity of the muscles most likely play a significant role in the formation of scoliosis and other spinal distortions. Busquet and others added a visceral theory to this. For the posturologists, the locomotor system, and the feet in particular, play an eminent role. Most likely, they are all correct.

The therapist should consider all three views and take them into account in the treatment plan. We must not forget here that the muscles always play an active role. **According to the law of function and structure, the muscles will adapt to the circumstances.**

Louisa Burns and other researchers have shown that this process begins very early. Therefore, you should never in the search for a cause disregard the treatment of the myofascial chains in cases of scoliosis. The same holds true for malpositions, whether they are the result of traumas or of excessive or misplaced strain in daily life.

8.4 Specific Characteristics of Some Muscles or Muscle Groups

Here we will not give a detailed account of anatomy, but limit ourselves only to the essentials and possible specifics of the following muscles and muscle groups:
- SCM
- Scalene muscles
- Diaphragm
- Iliopsoas
- Hip rotators

■ Sternocleidomastoid Muscle

The sternocleidomastoid muscle (SCM) (**Fig. 8.6**) consists of two muscle parts that attach caudally to the manubrium sterni and clavicles, and cranially to the superior nuchal line. Its cranial attachment lies on the occipitomastoid (OM) suture, which for Sutherland carried a special significance for cranial mobility. Restrictions of the OM suture limit the movements of the PRM. For this reason, the SCM is of particular significance.

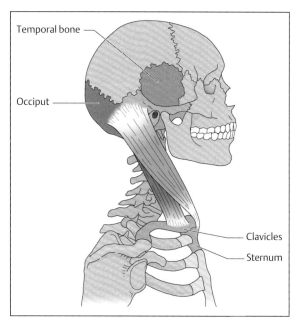

Fig. 8.6 Sternocleidomastoid muscle.

Functions
Bilateral
- Both SCMs together bend the CSC to pull the chin to the chest.
- In cases with hyperextended head, they pull the chin forward and help the neck muscles with the extension.
- They prevent the hyperextension of the CSC in a sudden push from behind, as, for example, in a whiplash trauma.
- They are inhalatory muscles.
- They are important for spatial orientation.

Unilateral
- In one-sided tension, the SCM bends the head and turns it to the other side, in the process of which the chin is lifted.
- Together with the trapezius, the SCM makes a pure sidebend.
- In scolioses, the SCM together with the trapezius straightens the head.

Innervation
- Accessory nerve
- CSC segments C1–C3

The SCM is a muscle with a tendency to shortening (postural muscle). Because of its course and the numerous adaptive options, it is difficult to compare the length of the SCM. Diagnosis is done by palpating the muscle for trigger points or indurations.

■ Scalene Muscles

The scalene muscles (**Fig. 8.7**) normally consist of three muscles: the scalenus anterior, scalenus medius, and scalenus posterior. Sometimes, a fourth muscle is present, the scalenus minimus. In most cases, though, it does not exist but is replaced by vertebropleural ligaments.

The scalenus anterior originates at the transverse processes of C3–C6 and attaches to the first rib, at the scalene tubercle.

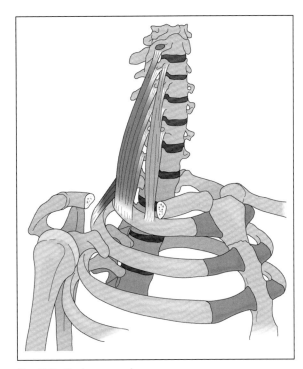

Fig. 8.7   Scalene muscles.

The scalenus medius originates at the transverse processes of C2–C7, to attach caudally at the first rib.

Between these two scalene muscles, we find the scalene hiatus or the "thoracic inlet," through which the subclavian artery and the brachial plexus pass. A spasm of the scalene muscles can irritate these structures.

The scalenus posterior attaches at the posterior tubercles of the transverse processes of C4–C6 and extends to the second rib.

The scalenus minimus, lastly, originates cranially at the anterior tubercles of the last two cervical vertebrae and runs to the pleural dome. The scalene muscles tend to spasms, but can also be affected by shortening and fibrosis. This depends on function. Trigger points can imitate the symptoms of neuralgia of the median nerve. The scalene muscles do for the CSC what the iliopsoas does for the LSC. They are primarily for bending the CSC, but can also assist in forming lordosis, if necessary. This ambivalent function perhaps explains their susceptibility to spasms.

Together with the longus capitis and longus colli, the scalene muscles belong to the prevertebral muscles. They are enclosed by the deep neck fascia and part of the Sibson's fascia that forms the upper thoracic diaphragm. As such, they have a connection to the central tendon and the visceral compartment.

Functions
Bilateral
- The frontal scalene muscles can flex the CSC.
- Together, they stabilize the CSC in the frontal plane.
- They are important muscles for inhalation. Electromyographic studies have shown that they become active together with the diaphragm. By pulling the upper thoracic aperture and therefore the pleural dome upward, they prevent the diaphragm from pulling the lungs caudally during inhalation. They are responsible for high thoracic respiration.

Unilateral
- Ipsilaterally, the scalene muscles are sidebenders of the CSC.

Innervation
- C3–C8

▪ Diaphragm

Still said something like this about the diaphragm (**Fig. 8.8**): "Through you, we live, and through you, we die" (Still's biography[140]). This is all the more true because the diaphragm in fact influences all vital functions:
- The gas exchange in the lungs is regulated by changes in pressure during inhalation and exhalation.

  Cellular metabolism is also activated by the pressure changes that induce respiration. During inhalation, a centrifugal pressure is created that is counteracted by the peripheral muscles. This produces rhythmic pressure changes that influence diffusion and osmosis. Inhalation sucks the blood towards the thorax. The abdominal organs are compressed; the venous sinuses of the skull and the neck veins are widened.
- The upward and downward movement of the diaphragm mobilizes all the organs in a rhythmic fashion, around their physiological movement axes.
- If necessary, the diaphragm assists in matters of posture. Changes in pressure conditions in the abdomen and chest can modulate the posture of the spinal column. Thereby, it can provide stability for the trunk and at the same time facilitate the movements of the extremities.
- Also of importance are the vascular and neural structures that pass through the diaphragm.

Because of its numerous functions, the diaphragm is in a dysfunctional state in every patient. The diaphragm separates the thoracic from the abdominal cavity and consists of two parts:

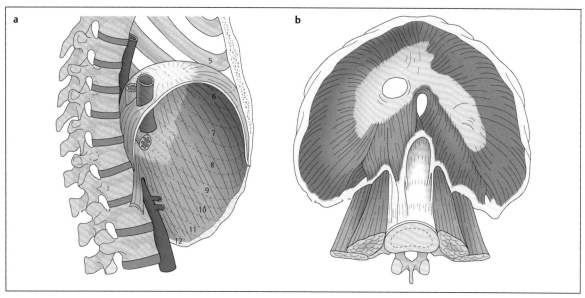

Fig. 8.8a, b Diaphragm.

- A fibrous part, the central tendon, to which organs attach
- A peripheral muscular part, which is responsible for its movements

The muscular part has attachments on the five last ribs and first three lumbar vertebrae. Nerves, vessels, and organs pass through openings of the diaphragm. The muscle fibers roughly run a course from cranial medial to caudal lateral, from the central tendon to the periphery.

Innervation
- Motoric: the two phrenic nerves (C3–C4–[C5]).
- Sensory: the central tendon is supplied by the two phrenic nerves, just like the dorsal part of the muscular part.
- The lateral muscle part is supplied sensorily from the segments T7 to T10.

Respiratory Movement and its Influence on the Locomotor System

The following muscles participate in respiration:

Inhalation
- Primary inhalatory muscles:
  - diaphragm
  - scalene muscles
  In rest position, only these two muscles are normally active.
- Accessory respiratory muscles:
  - SCM
  - trapezius
  - pectoralis major
  - pectoralis minor
  - quadratus lumborum
  - iliopsoas
  - serratus anterior
  - rhomboids
  - long back stretchers
  - intercostal muscles

The recruitment of these muscles depends on the depth of inhalation. First to be recruited are the intercostal muscles, from cranial to caudal.

During inhalation, the crus of the diaphragm pulls the central tendon down. This lowers the pressure in the chest, which leads to the inhalation of air. At the same time, pressure is increased in the abdomen and thereby also on the abdominal wall. These changes are proportional to the depth of inhalation.

The central tendon is moved downward until it is checked by pressure in the abdomen. After that, the costal fibers of the diaphragm pull the ribs upward. The thorax with sternum is raised. The diaphragm is supported in this process by the scalene muscles. The intercostal muscles stabilize the ribs against each other. In deeper inhalation, the other inhalatory muscles are also utilized.

The spinal column must be stabilized in order to lift the chest and widen the ribs. This is done by the iliopsoas and quadratus lumborum in the LSC and by the long back stretchers in the thoracic region.

The quadratus lumborum and the iliopsoas additionally stabilize the last two ribs and the upper LSC, by which the crus of the diaphragm gains a stable support.

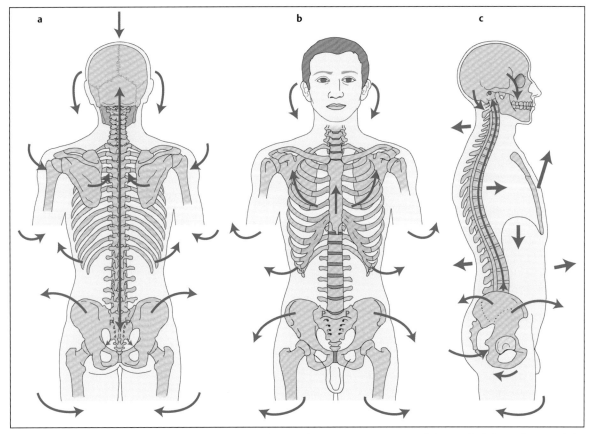

Fig. 8.9a–c   a, b Movements of the peripheral bones during inhalation. **c** Movements of the trunk skeleton during inhalation.

The shoulder blade fixators stabilize the scapula and give the serratus anterior and pectoral muscles the opportunity to raise the ribs.

The scalene muscles extend the cervical spinal column. At the end of a deep inhalation, the SCM is activated. It pulls the sternum up and prevents a flexion of the occiput, so that the gaze can continue to be directed straight ahead.

The abdominal muscles work eccentrically. They control the descent of the abdominal organs.

What happens to the pelvis, the cranium, and the extremities during inhalation? (See **Fig. 8.9**.)

The downward movement of the central tendon presses the abdominal organs downward and forward. This exerts pressure on the pelvic floor and abdominal muscles. The pressure on the pelvic floor pulls the pubic branches backward, the apex of the sacrum with the coccyx forward, and the ischiadic tubers medially. This pulls the iliac wings forward and outward. The pull of the pelvic floor on the coccyx mobilizes the basis of the sacrum dorsally into a contranutation. These movements are supported by the iliopsoas, which pulls the LSC into flexion and presses the pubic branches backward.

The pelvis also makes a movement, as we have described for the extension pattern. This conforms to the flexion movement of the craniosacral rhythm.

The lower extremities make a flexion–external rotation–abduction movement. The extension of the CSC and adduction of the shoulder blades rotate the shoulder joint outward. The flexion–abduction–external rotation of the shoulders is facilitated.

During inhalation, the upper thoracic aperture is raised. The cervical fascia is tightened like the roof of a tent. This pulls the temporal bones into external rotation. The SCM and trapezius muscles pull the occiput into extension, which corresponds to a craniosacral flexion.

The nuchal ligament supports these efforts passively. The extension of the CSC makes it taut. One way to avoid this pull is to pull the back of the head forward and downward, that is, into the cranial flexion.

The downward movement of the diaphragm and the resulting tension on the central tendon is neutralized by the elevation of the chest. This allows the SBS to move cranially.

Inhalation thus completely matches the flexion pattern of the PRM as described by Sutherland. The flexion stage is, like inhalation, an active stage. Exhalation is the opposite: a passive stage.

Exhalation

- The exhalation stage in rest is normally a passive process, in which the elasticity of the tissue returns the structures to their original position.
- In deep exhalation, it is mostly the abdominal muscles that are active. For some authors, the internal intercostal muscles are exhalatory muscles, as well as the transversus thoracis (Basmajian).

The diaphragm and the scalene muscles relax, just like the accessory respiratory musculature after having been activated in deep inhalation. In deep exhalation, the abdominal muscles become active. The content of the abdomen is compressed and pushed upward, while the chest is simultaneously pulled caudally.

In the ISJ, a posterior rotation of the ilium with an inflare occurs. The extremities make an internal rotation. The exhalatory position of the chest, via the ribs, pulls the upper TSC into flexion and the CSC into lordosis. The skull bones return into their original position. Compared with the position during inhalation, this corresponds to an extension–internal rotation. The position of the occiput corresponds to that of the sacrum.

Note: It is noteworthy that the head remains horizontal in both inhalation and exhalation. In our opinion, this is due to the associated action of the SCM, trapezius, and suboccipital muscles.

▪ Iliopsoas

The iliopsoas muscles (**Fig. 8.10**) might well be the most interesting muscles of the entire myofascial system. They are certainly the muscles whose functions are discussed with the most controversy. Because of their attachments and especially their course, they are able to adjust the position of the hip, pelvis, and LSC to each other.

For Basmajian, they are the most important muscles of the body for posture. They are able to adjust the spinal column and the pelvis in both the frontal and sagittal planes.

Lewit writes that the psoas often causes abdominal pain in the iliac fossa or imitates gall or renal colic.[86] The psoas is directly involved in respiration due to its origination in T12 and the medial arcuate ligament of the diaphragm.

Bogduk[14] states that a psoas spasm places enormous strain on the lumbar intervertebral disks. Fryette,[56] Kuchera,[82] Di Giovanni,[49] and others describe the psoas syndrome as the main cause for acute lumbago.

The psoas is considered a postural muscle; that is, a muscle with type-I fibers. We do, in fact, commonly find shortened iliopsoas muscles, but just as frequently spasmodic ones. According to Lewit,[86] a psoas contraction causes pain in the thoracolumbar junction (TCJ), and hypertonicity of the iliac causes pain in the ISJ.

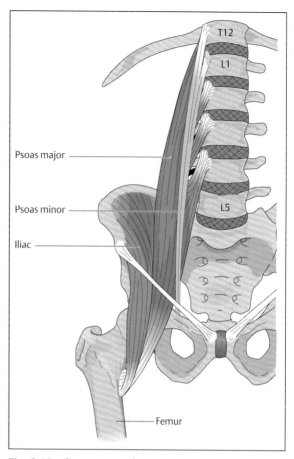

Fig. 8.10 Iliopsoas muscles.

Hypertonicity of the psoas can cause nerve irritations in the lumbar plexus. The psoas originates in the vertebral bodies T12–L4 (L5) and the intervertebral disks in between, as well as in the transverse processes of L1–L4. The lumbar plexus passes between the bellies of the two muscles. The iliac muscle has its origin in the iliac fossa.

Both muscles unite and run below the inguinal ligament to the lesser trochanter of the femur. The psoas minor originates at the belly of the psoas major and has a caudal attachment at the crista pectinea and the inguinal ligament.

The iliopsoas is enveloped by taut fascia, namely the iliac fascia. This is a caudal extension of the diaphragm fascia. The iliac fascia is connected at the pelvis with the inguinal ligament.

The muscle serves as slide rail for the kidney and is also in contact with the other organs. Its course is from dorsal–medial–cranial to caudal–ventral–lateral. At the level of the crista pectinea, the fibers change direction and run towards dorsal-lateral.

The muscle passes in front of the hip joint, from which it is separated by a bursa. This reversal in the direction of the fibers at the pubic ramus has the effect that the muscle turns the ilium ventrally when tensed. The psoas thereby supports the pull of the iliac.

Functions

Bilateral

- Both iliopsoas muscles are the strongest hip flexors in the body. With the legs stabilized, they turn the iliac wings forward and thereby create an anteversion of the pelvis. They are flexors of the lumbar vertebrae when the pelvis is prevented from tipping forward.

Unilateral

- They are ipsilateral side benders of the LSC. If the spinal column is able to form a lordosis at this point (is in "easy flexion" according to Fryette), the vertebrae turn into the convexity. If the pelvis is unable to tip forward (tension of the abdominal muscles or the pelvic floor), the psoas with the LSC make a flexion, sidebending, and ipsilateral rotation.

Innervation

Lumbar segments L1, L2 (L3)

▪ Hip Rotators

The muscle group of the hip rotators (**Fig. 8.11**) is formed by the piriformis, gemelli, obturator internus, and obturator externus. These are all muscles close to the joint, whose lever arm is too short to carry out strong movements. Therefore

they have more of a proprioceptive function for the hip joint. They adapt the rotation of the femur to that of the ilium, with the goal of centering the head of the hip optimally into the hip joint socket. In conjunction with the pelvic floor muscles, they form a sort of hammock for the pelvis.

In the stance stage of the gait and in one-legged stance, the piriformis and gluteus maximus stabilize the diagonal axis of the sacrum. The piriformis is a postural muscle that tends to shortening. It leaves the pelvis through the greater ischiadic notch. Here it is in close connection with the gluteal nerves, the pudendal nerve, the ischiadic nerve, as well as the vessels that supply the pelvic floor. Contraction of the piriformis can irritate these structures and cause pseudoneuralgias or disturbances in perineal function. The leg is then rotated outward and shortened. The pain radiates outward to the ISJ, the buttocks, and the backside of the thigh. In rare cases, the pain extends more deeply into the back of the knee. Longer sitting or squatting with knees pressed together causes pain because the piriformis is stretched (in the case of a piriformis lesion).

Functions

As already mentioned, hip rotators have a proprioceptive function for the hip joint. They are outward rotators for the hip and abductors, as well as light extensors. In hip flexions of over 60º, the piriformis serves as inward rotator of the hip.

We could continue this list of interesting muscles and muscle groups at will, but want to leave it at this. However, before concluding this chapter, we want to say a few words about the ventral muscles:

- The muscles of the hyoid bone play an absolutely minor role as mobilizers of the CSC. They are mainly active in movements of the lower jaw (mouth opener), whereby the lower muscles stabilize the hyoid bone. They play a role in swallowing, yawning, speaking, and breathing.

  Their main function lies most likely in preventing the collapse of the trachea and gullet during head and neck movements.

  To function as head flexor, the mouth has to be closed by the muscles of mastication.

  It is primarily the prevertebral muscles and the SCM that function as flexors of the CSC (when the head is flexed).

- The intercostal muscles stabilize the trunk and contribute to trunk rotations. In this aspect, they are synergists of the oblique abdominal muscles. Their main function, however, lies in assisting the respiratory muscles. This characteristic also holds true while they carry out support functions.

  The abdominal muscles, especially the rectus abdominis, are antagonists of the longissimus thoracis, a fact that emphasizes their affiliation with the thoracic muscles.

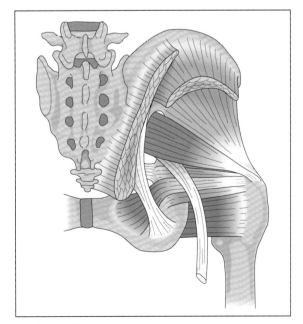

Fig. 8.11 Hip rotators.

They are active in almost all movements of the trunk and lower extremities. Herein, they act less as mobilizer than as stabilizer of the trunk, by compressing the abdominal organs and the thorax, which supports the spinal column.

The abdominal muscles and the lumbar multifidi muscles are active in gait before the muscles of the lower extremities (the transversus abdominis is the first).

With the exception of the hip rotators, all other muscles we have introduced (SCM, scalene, diaphragm, and iliopsoas) have the option to support other muscles in flexion as well as extension of the spinal column:

- The SCM extends the upper CSC and flexes it when the lower CSC is in flexion.
- The scalene muscles are benders of the CSC.
  When the paravertebral muscles in the neck make the CSC lordotic, the scalene muscles change their function to support the paravertebral muscles.

- The diaphragm can flex or extend the TCJ, depending on need.
- The iliopsoas can assist in making the LSC lordotic or extending it.
  When the abdominal muscles and pelvic floor retroverse the pelvis, the psoas makes the LSC kyphotic. The hip rotators are muscles whose significance is underestimated. During walking, the weight shifts from the sagittal to the frontal plane. Movement in the pelvis changes from a flexion–extension of the spinal column into an abduction–adduction (to maintain equilibrium). The hip rotators assist in stabilizing the pelvis and guarantee a good congruence of the hip ball in the joint socket. As a result, these muscles are frequently overloaded in all pelvic dysfunctions.

9 Posture

9.1 Hinge Zones

Osteopaths, chiropractors, and posturologists are equally aware of the significance of posture for the health of the organism. All three professions have different explanations for the causation of malpositions and similarly different approaches to treatment. They realize the significance of the spinal column, but find the main causes for imbalances in different regions of the body. Their treatment successes justify their methods.

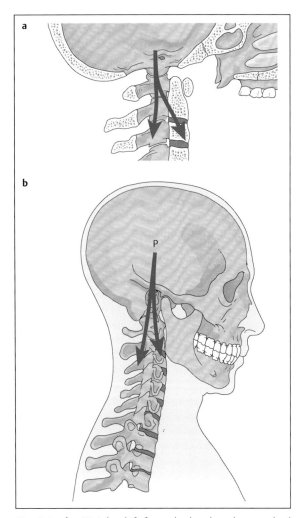

Fig. 9.1a, b Weight shift from the head to the vertebral body and the zygapophyseal joints of the axis (in the sagittal plane).

We asked ourselves why the osteopath considers the pelvis (and the occipitoatlantoaxial [OAA] complex), the chiropractor the atlas, and the posturologist the feet, as so important. What do these three areas have in common that has such a significant impact on posture? Not completely unexpectedly, we found a potentially interesting answer in anatomy or rather the biomechanics of these areas of the body.

The OAA complex, the iliolumbosacral junction, and the back foot have two important things in common:

1. In all three areas, we find a bone whose movements depend on the pressure exerted upon it. Direct mobilization by muscles is secondary:
   - The atlas acts like a meniscus between occiput and axis.
   - Globally, it acts opposite to the occiput and C2.
   - The sacrum makes movements that are opposite in relation to the spinal column and ilium. Pressure coming from the spinal column forces this action onto the sacrum.
   - The talus has no muscle attachments. Its behavior is solely dependent on pressure. The orientation of the malleolus fork and the position of the calcaneus impose movement directions onto the talus.
   - We can compare the behavior of these three bones with that of a ball in a ball-bearing.
   - The ball permits harmonious movements and makes it possible to shift pressure to another direction.
2. In all three areas, we find a redistribution of pressure conditions:
   - The weight of the body is distributed to the vertebral body and the zygapophyseal joints of C2 through the atlas (Mitchell: the facets of the cervical spinal column [CSC] have a weight-bearing function[107]) (**Fig. 9.1**).
   - At the lumbosacral junction (LSJ), gravity is shifted into a different plane.
   - From the sacral promontory, weight is transferred in the direction of the two hip joints (**Fig. 9.2**).
   - The talus distributes the body weight during standing and walking to the calcaneal tuberosity and in the direction of the cuboid and navicula, that is, to the outer and inner edge of the foot (**Fig. 9.3**).

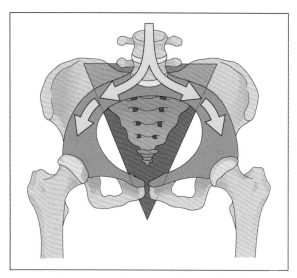

Fig. 9.2 Weight shift in the frontal plane from the spinal column into both hip joints.

Note: In these three areas, the redistribution of weight takes place in different planes:
- OAA: In the sagittal plane: facets and vertebral bodies of C2
- LSJ: In the frontal plane: in the direction of the two hip joints
- Foot: In the horizontal plane: from the talus to the calcaneus and the cuboid and navicula

This once again demonstrates the adaptation of structure to function. During walking, a posteroanterior weight shift occurs in the spinal column, from right to left and vice versa in the pelvis, and from the calcaneus to the metatarsal heads V and I in the foot.

Dysfunctions or structural changes in these areas cause these force transferences to be misdirected, which leads to additional strain on the muscles. Consequently, changed muscle pulls develop, as a result of which the entire locomotor system adapts and forms a different postural pattern.

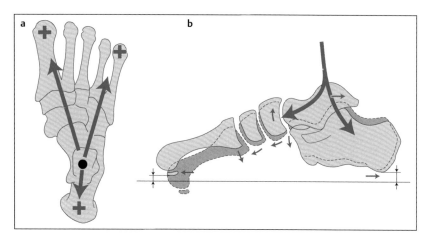

Fig. 9.3a, b Weight shift in the horizontal plane in the lower ankle joint.

9.2 Postural Balance

Posture is the result of musculoskeletal efforts to counteract the effects of gravity. Any deviation from the ideal posture coincides with heightened mechanical stress for the whole organism.

Kappler[74a] defines perfect posture as a state in which the mass of the body is distributed in such a way that the muscles maintain their normal tone and that ligamentous tensions neutralize the effect of gravity.

In standing people, posture depends primarily on three factors:
- On the evenness or unevenness of the ground upon which the person is standing
- On the state of the feet, as point of contact with the ground
- On the sacral base as pedestal for the spinal column, which keeps the organs of equilibrium plumb

Note: This holds true when we consider that a malposition of the OAA complex results in an adaptation of the sacrum. The OAA complex is bound to be balanced if the sacral base is horizontal. Nevertheless, we are inclined to add the OAA complex as a fourth factor because cranial dysfunctions can also be primary.

The three arches of the foot must be optimally balanced on both sides. The tibia should ideally stand perpendicular above the foot (in the frontal plane), so that the weight is distributed harmoniously onto the three arches. This guarantees an optimal transfer of force towards the pelvis. Here, we can already see the effects of uneven myofascial pulls on posture.

The iliolumbosacral junction is made up of the LSJ and the two iliosacral joints (ISJs). Stability is here ensured by the configuration of joints, by ligaments, and muscles. With optimally oriented forces, the joints are compressed in such a way that no muscle effort is required to stabilize the pelvis.

The base tone of the muscles and ligaments guarantees that the joint surfaces are congruent. The three forces that meet at the LSJ neutralize each other. The gravity that affects the sacral base is neutralized by the two rising forces from the legs. This mechanism functions only when the sacral base is horizontal. Even a minor inclination of the promontory changes the line of force and leads to instability. Consequently, muscles are recruited to ensure stability. This by necessity has a detrimental effect on the entire locomotor system. The position of the pelvis is changed, and thereby also the position of the spinal column and the lower extremities.

Robert Irvin determined in a study [in[155]] that people with chronic back pain who had received traditional osteopathic treatment but without lasting effects, experienced a 70% improvement of general symptoms when the sacral base was leveled by shoe inserts in addition.The most commonly found malpositions are:

- Flat feet (pes planus)
- Valgus of the back foot (pes valgus), pes abductus
- Lateral inclination of the sacral basis

All three of these deformities can be corrected with shoe inserts. Irvin found in a radiological study [in[155]] that 98% of all x-rayed persons had an average inclination of the sacral base of 1.2 mm in the frontal plane. A tilted sacral base (in the frontal plane) can have numerous causes:

- Sacral dysfunction: An anterior sacral base is also lower.
- Iliac dysfunction: The forward rotation of the ilium lifts the sacral base on the same side; a backward rotation lowers it on the same side.
- Leg length differences: Anatomical or acquired by traumas, surgeries, foot malpositions.

Adaptations of the spinal column to a tilted sacral base are always three-dimensional. The result can be a c-shaped (more rarely) or s-shaped scoliosis. Adaptation by an s-shaped curve is most economical. It facilitates the maintenance of equilibrium most easily. In newborns and toddlers, however, we only find c-shaped scolioses.

Rotation and sidebending are always opposite in cases with scoliosis and scoliotic posture (neutral position–sidebending–rotation [NSR] according to Fryette—see Chapter 3). Functional scoliosis (scoliotic posture) can develop into structural scoliosis (adaptation of structure to function).

The organism tries to compensate for disturbed posture by allowing the sections of the body above and below the disturbed area to adapt in the opposite direction. This leads to alternating rotation–sidebending. These changes develop in the transition zones.[82] The Zink patterns are an example of this (see Chapter 7): Littlejohn's model of the biomechanics of the spinal column supplies the mechanical explanation (see Chapter 5).

The treatment of scolioses or kypholordoses depends on whether the curves are functional or structural. In functional, not fixated curves, the goal is an improvement of posture. In the case of structural malposture, treatment aims primarily at alleviating pain and facilitating the optimal functioning of all structures and systems.

In each case, all possible causes of the malposition should be considered:

- Eyes
- Organs of equilibrium
- Cranium and OAA complex
- Temporomandibular joint
- Organs
- Spinal column/pelvis
- Feet

Fibroses, retractions, and adhesions must be treated specifically and over a longer time. Dynamic inserts are often very effective because they are able to stimulate those muscle chains specifically that are hypoactive. Furthermore, they are able to imitate a weight shift that influences the equilibrium via the vestibulospinal tracts.

It is often necessary, in structural changes of the feet to stabilize the foot arches with a postural shoe insert, in order to prevent nociceptive reflexes due to muscular overexertion. Leg length differences, whether anatomical or acquired, should be normalized when they are greater than 3 mm.[81]

9.3 Leg Length Differences

True leg length differences are common:
- 10% of humans have leg length differences of more than 1 cm.[145]
- Friberg (in [145]) examined 359 symptom-free soldiers radiologically and detected that:
  - 56% had leg length differences of 0–4 mm
  - 30% had differences of 5–9 mm
  - 14% had differences of 1 cm
- Two out of three chronic lumbago patients have radiologically proven leg length differences.

Leg length differences lead to a tilted sacral base with a compensation of the entire spinal column (rotoscoliosis). A tilted sacral base, on the other hand, regardless of its cause, always results in an iliac rotation, which in turn affects leg length. This is referred to as a functional leg length difference.

Before compensating for a difference in length with an insert, you have to find out whether you are dealing with a structural or functional difference. The only reliable method to detect this is an x-ray picture, after the somatic dysfunction of the whole organism has been treated. This is important because an iliac rotation results in a changed leg position, as a result of which the leg length can be changed up to 1 cm.[28] For this purpose, the pelvis and both legs have to be x-rayed in stance. The range of error in measurements in the x-ray pictures varies between 1–5 mm.[82]

▪ Postural Changes in the Pelvis and Spinal Column from Leg Length Differences

- The ilium on the side of the longer leg turns backward and that on the side of the shorter leg turns forward.
- The iliac crest is higher on the side of the longer leg.
- The entire pelvis tilts towards the shorter leg and rotates towards the longer leg.
- The sacral base tilts towards the shorter leg.
- The entire pelvis is anteriorized.
- The LSC lordosis is increased in most cases, especially at the LSJ.
- The LSC as a rule makes an NSR with rotation towards the short leg, the thoracic spinal column (TSC) an NSR towards the long leg, and the CSC a translation to the side of the short leg.
- The shoulder is lower on the side of the long leg, with the exception of cases in which the leg length difference exceeds 1.5–2 cm.
- The head tilts towards the side of the short leg.
- The pelvis makes a translation towards the long leg, as a result of which the lumbar triangle is greater on the side of the short leg.

Note:
- In ± 80% of cases, the LSC makes a sidebending movement to the long leg with an increase in the lordosis. In the other cases, it does not make any sidebending movement at all or one towards the short leg. This happens when structural damage prevents it from bending towards the long leg.
- Shoulder height is obviously influenced by the state of muscle tone in the trapezius and levator scapulae. A problem in the upper CSC can affect shoulder position.
- An iliac dysfunction affects leg length (functional leg length difference) and the position of the pelvic crest as well as that of the posterior superior iliac spine (PSIS) and anterior superior iliac spine (ASIS) in stance:
  - In a true leg length difference, the pelvic crest is higher, but the PSIS lower (depending on the difference in length) and posterior, the ASIS higher and posterior (dorsal rotation of the ilium).
  - In an ilium-anterior dysfunction, the crest is higher, but the PSIS higher on that side and the ASIS lower and anterior in comparison with the other side.
- In the first stage, the spinal column adapts with a global c-shaped scoliosis with inclination to the long leg. The entire musculoskeletal system, however, will react very quickly and establish an s-shaped curve. This distributes the stress and horizontalizes the eyes and organs of equilibrium.

▪ Effects on the Musculoskeletal System and Symptoms of Leg Length Difference

Most leg length differences remain asymptomatic until trauma or overexertion leads to pain symptoms. Even then, only the obvious differences are noted in most cases. Some patients report that they noticed that they have a "tilted pelvis" or that the public health physician already told them during a school examination that they have a spinal distortion.

Uncorrected leg length differences lead to myofascial tensions in the entire locomotor system. The LSJ is the area in which pain tends to manifest first. Later, the spinal column is affected up to the head. The myofascial tissue in the concavities is shortened, while it is stretched in the convexities.

Depending on what additional stress affects an area of the body, pain will manifest there when the adaptive mechanisms are exhausted.

In the LSJ, the iliolumbar ligaments are stretched on the convex side (short leg). This causes localized pain referring along the pelvic crest and in the groin, up to the inside of the thigh. We can frequently find a local tender point at the attachment of the ligaments to the pelvic crest or to the transverse processes of L4 or L5. The iliosacral ligaments on the same side are also frequently stressed. In addition to local pain, they can also produce pain on the lateral side of the thigh. Also common are tender trigger points on the quadratus lumborum, on the side of the LSC concavity. According to Lewit,[86, 86a] the scalene muscles on the same side are then hypertonic.

Rather common dysfunctions in the LSJ are a unilateral anterior dysfunction of the sacrum on the side of the short leg, or a forward torsion of the sacrum with rotation towards the long leg, as well as an extension–rotation–sidebending (ERS) dysfunction of L4 or L5.

In a posterior sacral torsion, the sacral base is generally posterior on the side of the long leg. Among the lower extremities, the long leg is most stressed mechanically. Here, we frequently find hip arthrosis, gonarthrosis (lateral tibia plateau), as well as muscular stress in the adductors, psoas, and gluteal muscles. A sciatica is more common on the side of the long leg (60%).

In leg length differences, we normally see a pronate position with valgus of the back foot on the long leg and an internal rotation of the leg. On the shorter leg, we more commonly find a supination of the foot. This explains why such patients wear out shoe soles on the outside more quickly on the side of the short leg.These phenomena are substantiated by different studies (all in [145]):

- Taillard and Morscher (1965): Electromyography (EMG) activity is increased in the erector spinae, gluteus maximus, and triceps surae on the side of the short leg.
- Strong (1966) found increased EMG activity in the muscles of the concavity in cases of scoliosis due to leg length difference, as well as in the postural muscles of the long leg.
- Bopp (1971) describes pain in the major trochanter, minor trochanter, the transverse processes of the lumbar vertebrae, and the pubis on the side of the long leg.
- Mahar et al. (1985): In a radiological study, they detected that an artificial lengthening of a leg causes an obvious pelvic shift to the side of the long leg.
- Wiburg (1983, 1984) describes the influence of a long leg on the hip joint. The pelvic shift towards the long leg decreases the pressure area on the hip joint, which causes increased pressure on the bones.

- Gofton and Trueman (1971) found in their research that 81% of patients suffering from hip arthrosis also had differing leg lengths, which affected the longer leg.

■ Diagnosis of a Leg Length Difference

A positive diagnosis of leg length differences of less than 1.5 cm difference in height at the pelvic crests can only be obtained radiologically. In such cases, it is recommended that the patient be treated osteopathically beforehand, that is, to normalize movement limitations and to treat the myofascial structures adequately to prevent these dysfunctions from distorting the picture. The error rate is still considerable.

Kuchera and Kuchera[82] therefore recommend subtracting 25% from the measured difference. Palpation and visual results can, however, give clear indication of leg length differences.The following clinical signs indicate leg length differences if they manifest concurrently:

- Pelvic crest and major trochanter are higher on the same side.
- PSIS and ASIS are higher on the side of the higher pelvic crest.
- PSIS dorsal and ASIS superior and dorsal on the side of the higher crest.
- With feet standing next to each other, we find a translation to the side of the long leg.
- The horizontal gluteal fold is higher on the side of the long leg.
- The lumbar triangle is greater on the side of the short leg.
- The shoulder on the side of the short leg is higher. Here we recommend palpating the lower shoulder blade angle.
- Pronate position of the foot of the long leg and supine position of the short leg.
- In leg length differences, the rest position is a weight shift to the short leg with a slight abduction and knee flexion in the long leg. Such people also frequently stand with legs spread apart.
- In maximum trunk bend, we find a higher inferolateral angle (ILA) on the side of the long leg.An examination with the patient lying down can also provide clues:
- In supine position with flexed knees, the knee is higher on the side of the long leg.
- In prone position with flexed knees, the thigh is longer (the knee further caudally) and/or the lower leg longer (heel higher) on the side of the long leg.

When most of these signs are present and the pelvic crests vary by 1 cm in height, you can assume that a leg length difference is present. This suspicion is strengthened when you ask the patient to walk and you realize that the pelvis is lifted on the side of the suspected longer leg during the swing stage of the gait, while the hip flexion is more obvious on the other side.

■ Should We Correct Leg Length Differences?

Kuchera writes[82] that recent studies prove that a sacral tilt of 1.5 mm affects the muscle tone of the LSC muscles and causes lumbago.

An interesting study was done by Klein, Redler, and Lowman.[76a] In 7 out of 11 children between 1.5 and 15 years of age, leg length differences completely normalized after compensating with shoes for 3–7 months. In this study, differences in length ranged from 1.3 to 1.9 cm.

Irvin (in [155]) writes that a complete correction of leg length difference—up to the point where the sacral base is horizontal—normalizes so-called idiopathic scolioses by one-third.

This indicates that shoe inserts are recommended when a true leg length difference (congenital or acquired) is present. The patient should at the same time also be treated with manual therapy to assist the organism in adjusting.

Differences of less than 3 mm are generally not corrected. Greater differences are corrected progressively. Irvin (in [155]) recommends an initial lift of 3 mm at most. Two weeks later, a further lift of 2 mm follows. In this way, the length of the leg is corrected every 14 days by 2 mm until the measured tilt of the sacral basis is completely evened out.

At the end of the entire procedure, the pelvis is again x-rayed and potential indicated corrections are performed. The pain disappears progressively from the pelvis up cranially.

If the required correction exceeds 8 mm, you should decrease the height of the shoe sole on the longer leg because an excessive one-sided correction changes the gait too much and can cause complications.

Kuchera[82] recommends correcting leg length difference of 5 mm and up with inserts. In greater differences, the tilt of the sacral base should be leveled by 50–75% of the radiologically measured difference (because we can assume a possible error in measurement of around 25%) with an insert or increase in shoe height. Hereby, the total condition of the patient and the duration of the imbalance must be taken into account:

- In patients with arthritic or osteoporotic bones or in labile patients, you should start with an increase of 2 mm, to which 2 mm are added in 2-week-intervals.
- In patients whose musculoskeletal state has not been affected substantially, you can begin with a build-up of 4 mm, to be increased by 2 mm every 14 days.
- In leg shortenings by trauma or surgery (prosthesis), the entire difference should be corrected at once.

An insert should not be thicker than 0.5 cm because it will otherwise cause discomfort in the shoe. If more build-up is needed, you can increase the shoe sole or lower the shoe sole on the long leg.

Because inserts on the heel alone result in pelvic rotation to the other side, it is recommended that the height in the entire sole be adjusted for any correction of 1.2 cm up. An insert under the heel or forefoot alone affects pelvic rotation. Because a leg length difference with tilted sacral base is often accompanied by a pelvic rotation (most commonly towards the long leg), it is frequently necessary to incorporate this aspect in the adjustment of shoe height. The reason is obvious: a pelvic rotation results in scoliosis in the spinal column:

- An insert under the heel turns the pelvis to the opposite side.
- An insert under the forefoot turns the pelvis to the same side.
- An even insert turns the pelvis to the same side because the insert under the forefoot has a greater effect than the insert under the heel.

In case of a leg length difference with pelvic rotation, the following rules of thumb apply for leveling out the sacral basis:

- Pelvic rotation of less than 5 mm: Traditional increase in shoe height according to the principles described above.
- Pelvic rotation between 5 and 10 mm: Begin with an increase of 3 mm under the forefoot and then in 2-week-intervals add 3 mm under the heel.
- Pelvic rotation greater than 10 mm: First correct the pelvic rotation with the insert, and afterwards increase both forefoot and heel with 3 mm each in 2-week intervals.

Note:
- For children, we recommend correcting a leg length difference with an insert because this increases pressure on the leg. This stimulates the lengthwise growth of the bones.
- Children should wear the insert until the leg length is evened out. Adults should use the inserts as regularly as possible.
- The procedures described above are general guidelines. They can be adjusted according to need.

◼ Conclusion

True leg length differences are very common. The literature states that 50–75% of the population have uneven legs. Studies in patients with chronic lumbago demonstrate that leg length differences are even more common here. In these cases, we are mostly dealing with differences of 5 mm or more.

More recent research seems to prove that a tilt of the sacral base of 1.5 mm affects the muscle tone in the lumbar region and can trigger lumbago. An improvement of symptoms by up to 80% (Kuchera[82]) due to leg length correction speaks for itself.

These facts emphasize the significance of posture in the case of back problems. Dysfunctions and traumas cause malpositions of the sacral base with predictable effect on the entire locomotor system. The fast adaptation of the myofascial tissue leads to rather fast structural changes, as a result of which the function of the entire organism is disturbed. A consequent osteopathic treatment has to take this fact into consideration and treat the myofascial tissue accordingly. The therapist who knows the physiology and pathophysiology of the myofascial tissue and muscle chains can treat specifically and give the patient precise instructions on which muscle groups to stretch and which ones to strengthen, with the stretching of shortened muscles preceding the strengthening of their antagonists.

10 Diagnosis

Before a patient can be treated, the therapist must perform a differentiated patient history and examination.

10.1 Medical History

The medical history is important for diagnosis by exclusion and is intended to provide the therapist with clues that are helpful in treatment. It should include questions about traumas, surgeries, and diseases and undergone treatments, as well as questions about the type, duration, and formative history of the symptoms. The therapist must furthermore get an idea about the patient's vegetative state.

10.2 Examination

The examination includes:
• Observation
• Palpation
• Motion tests
• Differential tests

▪ Observation

We observe the patient's posture in standing and supine position. Hereby, we register postural asymmetries, as well as muscle tensions and tissue changes. In stance, we can perform a series of global motion tests for individual regions of the body and evaluate these according to conspicuous features.

It is interesting to observe how patients assume their natural stance and then how they stand with their feet closely together. By reducing the basis for their equilibrium, we force them to clarify their postural pattern.

In the supine position, the factor of gravity is excluded. The motion pattern that now becomes visible is a manifestation of muscular imbalances as a result of dysfunctions (or structural changes).

Note: We are not strong proponents of a large-scale gait analysis. Frequently, the size of the clinic is not appropriate, and it is too time-consuming for the clues that it supplies, which are often quite minor. Rather, we prefer to analyze the gait through the hip-drop test, the single-leg stance, and shoulder movements.

▪ Palpation

Palpation gives the therapist clues to the position of the structures on the one hand, and to the condition of the tissue on the other. In addition to observing the posture in standing and lying position, palpation can provide clues about dominant muscle chains and the position of joint partners. Furthermore, it can facilitate a differentiation between chronic and acute processes. These findings are substantiated by motion tests.

▪ Motion Tests

Global motion tests serve to make the bodily regions with the most obvious limitations of movement stand out. In the trunk bend and sidebend (**Fig. 10.1**), we look for harmonious execution of movement. Interruptions or evasive movements are then examined in greater detail.

This area is examined with segmental tests and palpation for muscular or segmental restrictions. Based on differential tests, we finally attempt to find out whether it is the visceral, cranial, or parietal aspect of the problem that dominates in this patient. The part of the area that has been evaluated as dominant based on the findings is then treated specifically with adequate techniques.

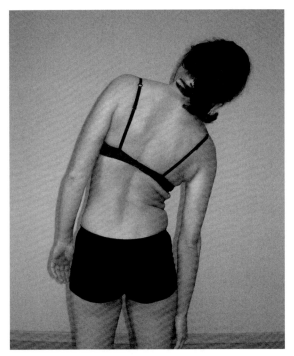 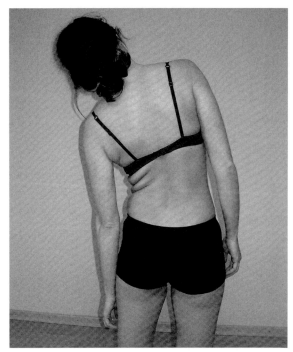

Fig. 10.1a, b Sidebending test for the lumbar spinal column.

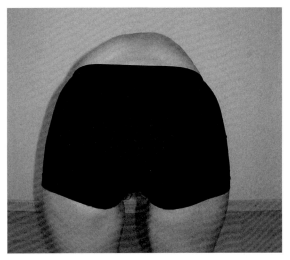

Fig. 10.2 Flexion test.

We would now like to introduce a slightly different, but very rational type of examination. It is based on the Zink patterns and a traction test at the head, pelvis, and legs.

After quickly observing the patient's posture in stance and registering rough deviations, we have the patient bend forward and perform the hip-drop test or a translation test at the pelvis. This gives clues about the position and mobility of the sacrum and lumbar spinal column, as well as potentially about a dominant muscle chain.

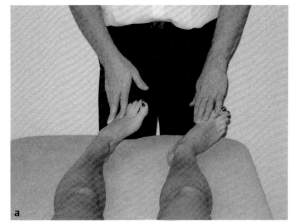

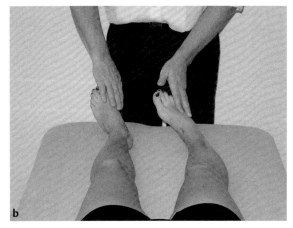

Fig. 10.3a, b Rotation test of the hip in side comparison.

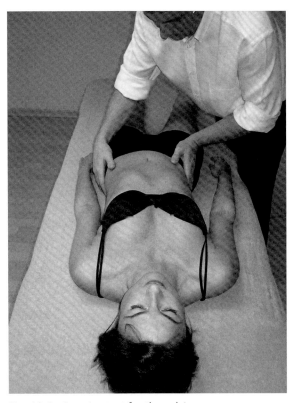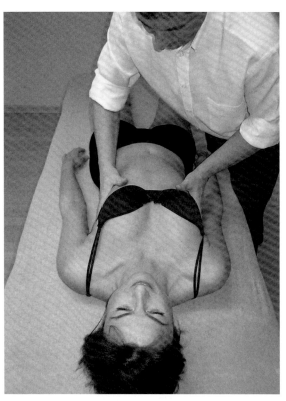

Fig. 10.4 Rotation test for the pelvis.

Fig. 10.5 Rotation test for the lower thoracic aperture.

If we find conspicuous features in the lower extremities, we have the patient do a single-leg stance. Here, we observe the behavior of pelvis, knees, and feet. Neuromuscular disturbances in the leg muscles manifest in postural asymmetries due to muscular imbalances and the different behavior of the receptors as a result of segmental "facilitation."

The flexion test (**Fig. 10.2**) can give clues about a dominant chain on the leg and in the spinal column. The hip-drop test and the translation test give information about the position of the sacrum and the lower LSC.

In the supine position, we observe the rotation of the hips (**Fig. 10.3**), legs, pelvis (**Fig. 10.4**), and the lower (**Fig. 10.5**) and upper (**Fig. 10.6**) thoracic apertures (LTA and UTA), before testing the Zink patterns. Afterwards, a traction test is performed at the head and pelvis (or in the legs) to allow us to find the dominant side. In addition, this test helps in localizing the primary restriction and in differentiating between ascending or descending chains.

The earlier resistance occurs in traction, the closer we know the dominant motion limitation in the traction hand to be.[137, 148]

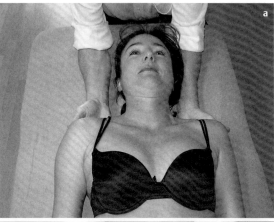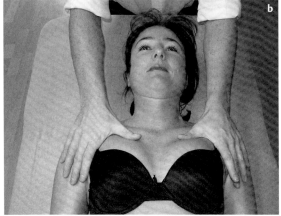

Fig. 10.6a, b Rotation test: (**a**) for the upper thoracic aperture (**b**) variation.

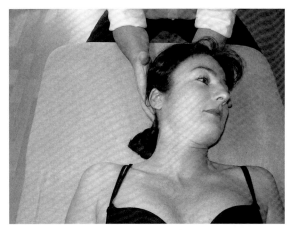

Fig. 10.7   Rotation test of the head joints (OAA).

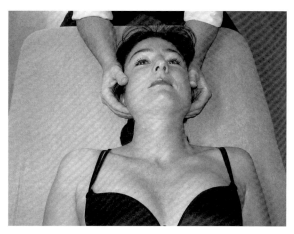

Fig. 10.8   Translation test of the atlas joint.

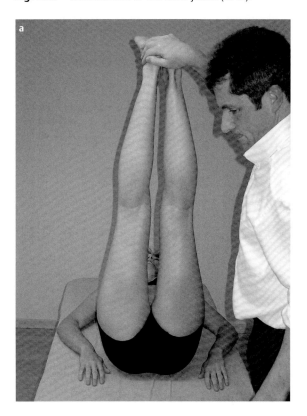

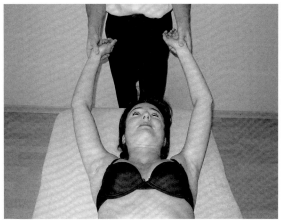

Fig. 10.9a, b   a Test for the ischiocrural muscles (hamstrings). The ischiocrural musculature is shortened on the left, as a result of which the ischiadic tuber is elevated. **b** Variation.

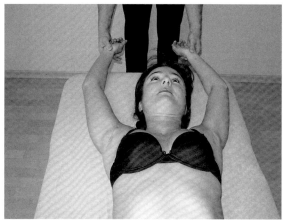

Fig. 10.10   Test of the pectoralis.

Fig. 10.11   Test of the latissimus dorsi.

In the Zink patterns, we not only test the torsions in the junctions to find out where they do not alternate, but also mainly attempt to detect the junction at which the rotation pattern manifests most obviously, that is, where the rightward rotation (**Fig. 10.12**) distinguishes itself most clearly from the leftward rotation. Subsequently, we differentiate whether these are dorsal or ventral muscles that form the torsion pattern.

Each junction represents a certain body region. We have presented this in the previous chapters. There are anatomical (muscles) as well as neurological interconnections that illustrate this (**Figs. 10.7–10.11**). Here, we provide another quick summary:

Occipitoaltlantaoaxial

• Suboccipital muscles
• Segments C1–C3

Upper Thoracic Aperture

• Sibson fascia
• Segments C4–T4

Lower Thoracic Aperture

• Diaphragm, abdominal muscles, and ribs VI–XII
• Segments T5–T12

Pelvis

• Psoas, pelvic floor
• Segments L1–S4

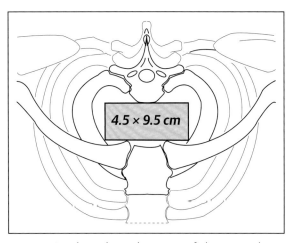

Fig. 10.12 The rightward rotation of the upper thorax aperture can be caused by ventral muscles on the left or by dorsal muscles on the right.

11 Therapy

Once we have found a predominant pattern, we need to examine in more detail all structures that are segmentally (neurally) connected with it, to direct therapy as specifically as possible, according to Still's principle: "find it, fix it, and leave it alone."

From our osteopathic perspective, the myofascial structures play a significant role:
- In acute, painful cases, we regularly find active trigger points. These frequently cause so-called "pseudo-neuralgias."
  Example: Trigger points in the scalene muscles imitate a medianus neuralgia. Trigger points in the gluteus minimus present with symptoms like an L4 ischialgia.

- So-called "silent trigger points" affect the normal behavior of the muscles and cause muscular imbalances.
- Retractions and fibroses in the muscles are often partial triggers of relapses.

If the therapist has found and treated (viscerally, parietally, or cranially) the dominant dysfunction, and in addition treats the trigger points in acute cases and normalizes the shortened musculature in the affected muscle chain in chronic cases, the chances are quite good that the painful state is relieved quickly and that the danger of relapses is reduced.

11.1 Muscle Energy Techniques

Muscle energy techniques (METs) are rather popular with manual therapists. Whether physiotherapist, chiropractor, osteopath, or manual therapist, they all employ muscle energy techniques or variations thereof to relax or tone muscles, to mobilize joints, or to stretch fasciae. Perhaps they are so popular because they are not dangerous and often successful even when applied inaccurately. It is possible that Kabat was the first therapist who treated spasms and muscle shortenings with muscle techniques.

Osteopaths credit Mitchell Sr. with the development of muscle techniques in the treatment of joint dysfunctions. The osteopathic community took note of this method after he composed two articles on manipulative treatments of mechanical dysfunctions in the pelvis with METs. Mitchell himself was influenced in the development of his method by the work of other osteopaths (T.J. Ruddy and Carl Kettler). Furthermore, he invoked Still himself who had stated that attempting to restore joint integrity before normalizing muscles and ligaments is like putting the cart before the ox.

Over the years, METs have been refined considerably by testing their efficacy in studies and taking into consideration the neurophysiological properties of the myofascial structures.

It is likely that other professionals (physiotherapists, chiropractors) have worked on the development of muscle techniques parallel to the osteopaths. Significantly, a lively exchange and encounters take place today between the leaders in the different fields. These include therapists like Mitchell Jr., Stiles, Greenman, Liebenson, Lewit, Janda, Grieve, and Norris, to name just a few. This could be the reason for the scientific progress in this subject.

▪ Definition

METs are defined as a form of osteopathic treatment in which the therapist asks the patient to tense a muscle from a closely controlled position in a specific direction against the precise resistance of the therapist.

METs are employed for the following purposes:
- To treat limited mobility in joints
- To stretch hypertonic muscles and fasciae
- To stimulate local circulation
- To change muscle tone with neuromuscular mechanisms

METs require the cooperation of the patient in tensing the muscle, breathing in or out, or in moving a joint partner in a certain direction. For these reasons, this form of therapy cannot be utilized with comatose, uncooperative people or patients who are unable to follow the therapist's instructions.

▪ Indications and Contraindications

Indications and contraindications are based on this definition of METs. The **indications** are varied. The following list does not by any means reflect an evaluation:
- Inhibiting hypertonic, spastic muscles
- Toning hypotonic, weak muscles
- Stretching fibroses, shortenings
- Releasing adhesions
- Normalizing joint dysfunctions
- Stimulating the local venolymphatic circulation
- Relieving pain
- Positively affecting motion and postural patterns
- Interrupting a pain-inducing vicious circle

In addition to the classic **contraindications** for osteopathic treatment, these also include:
- Communication and coordination problems between therapist and patient
- Bone or muscle injuries in the segments to be treated that have not yet healed

▪ Prerequisites for Optimal Muscle Energy Technique Application

1. One of the most important prerequisites is an accurate diagnosis. The therapist should be able to detect what triggers the pain, limits the movement, or is the cause of the imbalance or incorrect motion pattern.

Example:
- A painful shoulder–neck region can have many causes, which nevertheless all lead to muscular changes:
  - joint blockage in the CSC
  - trigger points
  - problems with the intervertebral disks
  - reflexive pain
  - ligamentous pain after trauma
  - hypertonicity or spasms as a reaction to postural or functional overexertion due to a shortening of other muscle groups

The treatment focus and choice of muscle energy technique differs for each of these causes!
- A limited hip extension can:
  - stem from the hip joints (beginning or advanced arthrosis)
  - be the result of a chronically shortened iliopsoas
  - be the result of a spastic shortened iliopsoas (in LSC disorders)

An attentive diagnosis will show the therapist whether the main problem lies in the muscle, fascia, or joint (that is, which of the three aspects dominates, because all three are often present).

For the therapy to be as efficacious as possible, it must specifically affect the element that triggers the pathomechanism. This applies to diagnostic techniques as much as to treatments.

2. It is important that the neurovegetative state of the patient is evaluated correctly. Typical examples are fibromyalgia patients, depressed people, and patients with acute pain. In such cases, the proper dose at the proper moment in the correct area of the body is key for the therapeutic progress.
3. The choice of treatment technique is significant. The technique must be able to target the lesion mechanism specifically; it must match the neurovegetative state of the patient; it must not be painful; and it should ideally show immediate measurable success.
4. Precision of the intervention.
5. To fulfill the requirements listed above, the therapeutic technique must exactly and to the appropriate degree affect the targeted joint, relax hypertonic or spastic muscle fibers, or stretch shortened fascia in the right direction.

▪ Technical Prerequisites and Enhancers for Muscle Energy Techniques

Therapists must have a good sense of touch, as well as the ability to distinguish between acute and chronic dysfunctions. They must be able to feel the affected muscle fibers in a hypertonic muscle. They must sense in which direction to stretch the muscle and when the muscle fibers react to the stretch.

For the treatment of joints with METs, it is important that the therapist senses the barriers in the three planes of movement and adjusts the joint partner correctly without stretching the muscles that are to be treated (to avoid the stretch reflex). Herein it is essential that they feel the muscular barrier. This is reached before the joint barrier and before the fascial barrier!

In general, joint restrictions are resolved before treating muscles or fasciae. This applies particularly in cases where the blocked joint has triggered muscular hypertonicity. In other cases, however, it is necessary to relax the muscles first before you can treat the joints.

The patient must be able to follow the instructions of the therapist. More than anything, the therapist must be able to relax and sense the difference between contraction and relaxation. The patient should be able to contract to the desired degree.

Of assistance are respiration, eye movement, and visualization:

Respiration

- Inhalation facilitates contraction, exhalation lessens it.
- It is helpful when the patient "breathes into the area" that is being treated.
- Inhalation should be slow and progressive.
- First, the patient should tense the muscles before then inhaling.

Eye Movement

This is particularly important for the treatment of the cervical spinal column (CSC). In general, the patient should look into the direction into which they contract.

Visualization

A mental image of the movement makes contracting and relaxing easier for the patient.

■ Variations of Muscle Energy Techniques

Before describing the different kinds of MET, we would like to introduce a few terms:

Isometric contraction: The distance between origin and attachment of the muscle does not change during contraction. The forces of the therapist and patient neutralize each other.

Isotonic concentric contraction: The muscle shortens during the contraction. The patient overcomes the resistance of the therapist.

Isotonic eccentric contraction: Muscle length is increased in spite of the contraction. Muscle fibers are stretched.

Physiological principles: The following physiological principles are utilized:

Postisometric relaxation: After contraction, a muscle relaxes more easily. During the relaxation phase, the previously tensed fibers can be stretched better. The relaxation phase must not be equated with the latent time, which is much shorter.

We suspect an activation of the golgi sensory system, which leads to an inhibition for 10–15 seconds. During this relaxation phase, the muscle group is stretched exactly until a new contraction occurs.

Reciprocal innervation or antagonist inhibition: The contraction of agonists relaxes their antagonists (in this motion pattern). This serves as foundation for the different variations of MET.

Muscle Strengthening

So-called isokinetic contractions during ± 4 seconds in a range of motion corresponding as much as possible to the motion pattern. The contraction should be close to maximal. Both concentric and eccentric contractions are performed. Short series of contractions are preferred to frequent repetitions.

Isolytic Muscle Energy Technique

This form of MET is utilized when you want to stretch a muscle or resolve adhesions. It involves an isotonic eccentric contraction. To break down as much fibrotic muscle fiber as possible, muscle contractions have to be correspondingly strong. This demands a rather large effort on the part of the therapist because they have to stretch the contracting muscle. Hence, we recommend pre-stretching the muscle until the therapist feels the tension in the fibers that are to be treated. If the therapist now asks the patient to contract, less strength is required.

Muscle Energy Technique for the Release of Spasms or Hypertonicity

For this purpose, isometric contractions are most suitable. Both PRI and antagonist inhibition can be utilized. The two methods can also be combined. It is important to stretch the muscle or muscle group only up to the muscular barrier. The required effort should not exceed 20% of the maximal contraction.

A contraction that is just barely felt in the hypertonic fibers is best. The hypertonic fibers are those muscle fibers that contract first during strain. Deciding between PRI or antagonist inhibition depends on the level of pain in the hypertonic muscle.

When the principle of antagonist inhibition is applied, the contraction can be greater. The decisive effect in this technique results from the passive stretch. This must be completely painless.

Joint Normalization by Muscle Energy Technique

Here again, both methods are applied. While ilium lesions are primarily treated by antagonist inhibition, we correct joint dysfunctions mainly with the principle of postisometric relaxation (PIR). In either case, isometric contractions are preferable.

Since we are mostly trying to inhibit postural (type-I) muscle fibers here, it is recommended that light contractions are maintained a little longer (5–7 seconds).

Treatment with muscle energy techniques can quickly and cause slight numbness in the treated area for ± 24 hours. This is most likely caused by the release of waste products in the tissue.

In cases of muscular imbalances, the hypertonic or shortened muscles must be stretched before the weak hypotonic muscles can be strengthened. Janda explains this with the principle of antagonist inhibition.

11.2 Myofascial Release Techniques

Paula Scariarti and Dennis J. Dowling [in [49]] also refer to myofascial release techniques as "myofascial tendon ligament osseous viscera techniques." This is an indication of the interrelations that the connective tissue forms between the individual systems.

Still's writings demonstrate that he accorded great significance to the connective tissue. It is most likely he also utilized myofascial relaxation techniques. The Still techniques that are taught by Van Buskirk[23] are the best evidence for this. Myofascial release techniques aim at relaxing the connective tissue.

When we consider the fact that the connective tissue is composed of muscles, skin, fasciae, tendons, ligaments, capsules, serous membranes, mesoderm, and so on, treatment takes on a holistic shape.

The terms "tight/loose" and "direct/indirect" as well as the "three-dimensionality" are significant during diagnosis and treatment:

Loose/Tight

These terms describe the two extreme states of the tissue. Both are pathologic and contribute to imbalances. If a muscle or muscle group is hypertonic or shortened, it is tight. Its antagonist then tends to be hypotonic or loose.

The myofascial release technique aims at restoring balance through neuromuscular and mechanical reflexes, to support the physiological functions.

Direct/Indirect

These terms are significant in treatment. In direct treatment, the tight tissue is tensed even more. This activates receptors in the tissue, which then cause relaxation. The other method consists of approximating the tensed tissue. This reduces tension and calms the receptors.

Both techniques require a good sense of touch. Most fasciae consist of tissue in which the fibers are not oriented unidirectionally but in different directions.

In direct treatment, we palpate continuously in the direction the tension manifests in. In indirect treatment, we follow the "relaxations" throughout the course of treatment.

Three-dimensional

For treatment as well as for the examination, we sound out the mobility of the tissue in all three planes. Depending on the treatment variation, relaxation (ease) and contraction (bind) are then stacked on top of each other. Both hands of the therapist are active, to palpate and to treat. For treatment, it is recommended to utilize so-called "enhancers":
- Respiration
- Movements of the extremities
- Eye movements
- Combinations of these three enhancers

Depending on the selected treatment variety, the enhancers are used to support either the direct or the indirect treatment form.

Clinical Procedure

The patient sits or lies on the back or on the abdomen. With both hands, the therapist palpates the area that is to be treated. The therapist tests the mobility of the tissue with both hands, as well as the tension between both hands in all planes. When tensions are found, the therapist must decide on a treatment variation. For indirect treatment, the therapist moves the hands in the free movement directions to approximate the tissue.

During the course of treatment, the movement directions change. The therapist follows each of the new directions. When the fasciae are to be treated directly, tension is built up between the hands by palpating the fascial trains in the three motor planes with both hands.

The tissue is kept under tension until the therapist detects harmonious craniocaudal movement or clearly feels the patient's breathing under the hands. Inhalations and movements of the extremities can help to increase the build-up of tension. In this context, it is interesting when the patient "breathes into" the area that is being treated. When the patient performs movements of the extremities, the therapist has to give instructions on which movements build or reduce tension. The patient should then perform the movements accordingly.

There are a number of other treatment methods that are based on the same principles as the myofascial release technique. We only list these treatment methods here without describing them in greater detail:
- Strain–counterstrain
- Facilitated positional release
- Functional techniques
- Balanced ligamentous release
- Unwinding
- Cranial osteopathy

11.3   Neuromuscular Technique

Neuromuscular technique (NMT) is an interesting myofascial treatment method. It involves deep massage of the muscles, performed with one or several fingers or the edge of the hand. The technique was developed in the 1940s by Stanley Lief, when he originally tried to develop a method for treating the tissue before a manipulation.

Lief was a chiropractor and osteopath. He was convinced that joint problems were only a partial cause for diseases, neuralgias, and circulatory problems, as the chiropractors believed back then. Furthermore, it was obvious to him that blockages in the spinal column are also often the result of induration of the paravertebral tissue. As a result, he began to massage the muscles sensitively with increasingly deep pressure. Hereby, he paid attention to knots, retractions, swellings, and resistances in tissue mobility.

He was quite surprised that he not only resolved movement limitations with this neuromuscular treatment, as he called his method, but it also had distal effects. He called his technique "neuromuscular treatment" because he was able to treat the muscles, but also reflexively via neural pathways—as he believed—influence other disorders.

Treatment effects do in fact appear to be primarily reflexive. This treatment method allows us to effectively treat trigger points, Chapman reflex zones, as well as other reflex points. On the other hand, it is possible by deep massage to specifically target and affect the connective tissue, to stimulate local circulation, and thereby to activate metabolism. This treatment can be applied to the whole body or only to certain areas.

Clinical Procedure

- The patient sits or lies as comfortably as possible.
- The finger is pressed into the tissue until the therapist can sense light resistance but without causing pain.
- The finger is then moved forward with a speed of ± 2–3 cm/sec:
  - When encountering indurations, knots, or resistance, the movement of the finger is slowed down without changing pressure.
  - As a rule, strokes of 5–10 cm in length are performed in this way.
  - In hardened areas, several strokes are performed until the tissue is softened.
  - In knots, frictions or intermittent pressure can be applied.
  - The strokes can run across or parallel to the muscle fibers.
  - Trigger points must generally be treated separately (see Part B, Trigger Points).

11.4   Myofascial Release Technique with Ischemic Compression

This refers to an interesting treatment of muscle indurations and trigger points.

Procedure

- The patient sits or lies relaxed.
- The therapist searches for indurations, hypertonic fibers, or trigger points in the muscles.
- The point, which is most often very painful (when pressed firmly), is compressed with the elbow or knuckle of the hand.
- The patient is instructed to make movements that will move the affected muscle fibers back and forth under the knuckle or elbow.
- Contact is maintained until the pain in the point is clearly lessened.
- Afterwards, the concerned muscle or muscle group is passively stretched several times.

B

Trigger Points
and Their Treatment
Eric Hebgen

12 Definition

A **trigger point** (TP) is a strongly irritated area within a hypertonic strand in a skeletal muscle or muscle fascia. The trigger point is painful upon touch and can cause point-specific referred pain, muscular tension (in other muscles as well), or vegetative reactions.

Trigger points also occur in other tissue, such as the skin, fatty tissue, tendons, ligaments, joint capsules, or periosteum. These trigger points are, however, not as constant and always localized identically as the myofascial trigger points. Furthermore, they do not cause referred pain.

13 Classification of Trigger Points

13.1 Active and Latent Trigger Points

Distinction is made between active and latent trigger points. Active trigger points cause pain, in rest as well as during muscular activity. Latent trigger points, by contrast, can show all the diagnostic signs of an active trigger point (see below), but only generates pain during palpation.

Active trigger points can transform into latent ones, especially when the factors that perpetuate the trigger point are lacking, or when the muscle is stretched sufficiently during normal daily activity.

Conversely, latent trigger points can persist silently for years in a muscle and then be transformed into active trigger points. Such a change may be facilitated for example, by excessive stretching or use of the muscle, that is, the dysfunction of muscular overexertion in the widest sense.

13.2 Trigger Point Symptoms and Supporting Factors

▪ Symptoms

The following symptoms suggest active or latent trigger points:
- Limited active and/or passive mobility in lengthening (stretching) or shortening of the affected muscle. A significant stiffness in movement may be felt.
- Weakness of the affected muscle
- Referred pain in characteristic patterns that are defined for each muscle. In active trigger points, the referred pain occurs during activity, rest, or palpation of the point. Latent trigger points form the typical pattern only during diagnostic palpation.

Muscular stiffness and weakness are especially noticeable after longer rest periods or generally after inactivity. Typical examples are morning stiffness or the muscular start-up pain after prolonged sitting.

The manifestation of symptoms and palpatory sensitivity of active trigger points can change within hours or from day to day. The symptoms of trigger point activity can outlast the triggering cause by a long time.

Other symptoms that can be caused by trigger points include:
- Vegetative changes in the zone of the referred pain, such as local vasoconstriction, sweating, increased lacrimal and nasal secretion, increased pilomotoric activity (goose bumps).
- Disturbed depth sensitivity
- Disturbance of equilibrium, vertigo
- Change in motorneuron activity with increased irritability
- Impaired muscular coordination

▪ Supporting Factors

Factors that support the formation of trigger points include:
- Acute muscular overstrain
- Chronic overwork with excessive tiring of the muscle
- Direct trauma
- Under-cooling (muscular activity without previous warm-up)
- Other trigger points
- Disease of the internal organs
- Arthritic joints
- Segmental reflectory dysfunction (see Chapter 18)
- Negative stress (distress)

14 Pathophysiology of Trigger Points

14.1 Locally Increased Tension in Trigger Points and Referred Pain

The local increase of tension in the trigger point is explained by a change, that is, increase in sensitivity of type-III and type-IV nerve fibers. These nerves—in the form of free nerve endings—make up the nociceptors in a muscle. When such a nerve fiber is sensitive to irritation, this means that even small stimuli, in this case pain stimuli, cause an amplified reaction in the body. The reaction can lead, for example, to a greater perception of pain or a more pronounced vegetative reaction. In general terms, a stronger reaction of the afferent nociceptive nerve fibers to a stimulus can cause efferent answers in nerves that would not react under normal circumstances. The processing of information for these phenomena takes place at the level of the segmental spinal cord.

Substances that are known to increase sensitivity in type-III or type-IV nociceptor fibers are, for example, bradykinin, serotonin, prostaglandin, or histamine.

Afferent impulses from type-III or type-IV nociceptor fibers can also be responsible for the fact that the brain "misinterprets" these impulses and responds with referred pain or increase in tension. The mechanisms responsible for this include the following:

14.2 Causes of Locally Increased Tension in Trigger Points and Referred Pain

■ Convergence Projection

Two alternative connections in which afferences are switched over to the efferent neuron exist in the bone marrow:
- An afferent nociceptive impulse from the skin and muscle or an internal organ is switched to one interneuron in the bone marrow that is responsible for both afferences, before this neuron is again switched to the efference, to respond to the stimulus.

- Skin, muscle, and visceral afferences have a shared end path, before the stimulus is conducted to the efference.

Afferent information is not only conducted to the efference to respond to the stimulus, but also through the spinothalamic tract into the central nervous system (CNS). As the afferent stimulus reaches it, the CNS is unable to distinguish whether the nociceptive impulse comes from the skin/muscle or an internal organ (**Fig. 14.1**). Because our body, or rather the CNS,

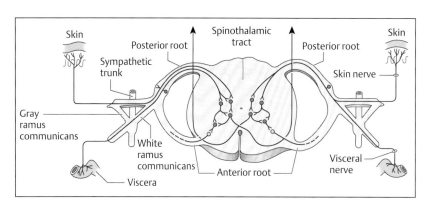

Fig. 14.1 Formative paths of transmitted pain.

has learned in the course of life that nociceptive, that is, harmful irritations generally hit the body from the outside, they are interpreted as coming from the skin or muscle: a pain stimulus that has been passed on for conscious perception through the spinothalamic tract is recognized as pain referred from the segmentally associated skin.

Afferent impulse activity from a trigger point is treated by the CNS like a nociceptive afference from an internal organ: The perception of pain takes place in the skin, that is, in the segmentally associated reference zone.

◾ Convergence Facilitation

Many afferent nerves carry out a background activity. We can say that they generate a type of base noise, an impulse activity that does not stem from external (or internal) stimuli, but has to be explained neurophysiologically as a lowered stimulus threshold due to changes in the ion channels. Consequently, action potentials are more likely to be triggered. This can be considered as a protective mechanism towards nociceptive stimuli that can therefore be recognized and responded to more quickly.

If such background activity in an area of the skin is heightened (convergence-facilitated) by a series of afferent nociceptive stimuli from an internal organ or trigger point and conducted to a neuron of the spinothalamic tract into the CNS (see Convergence Projection above), the pain is then perceived as very strong in that area of the skin.

◾ Axonal Ramifications

The dendrites of afferent nerves can branch out into diverse directions so that different areas of the body are captured sensitively by this nerve. This can result in the misinterpretation of an afferent stimulus by the CNS: the individual regions of the body can no longer be differentiated from the axon mound—as a consequence, the pain is perceived as stemming from the entire area that is innervated by the neuron.

◾ Sympathetic Nerves

It is possible that these nerves help in sustaining the referred pain by releasing substances that further sensitize the nociceptive afferences of the pain area and lower their stimulus threshold. It is also conceivable that sympathetic innervation causes the blood supply of the afferences from the pain area to be reduced.

◾ Metabolic Derailment

The trigger point zone is an area of the muscle that is characterized by metabolic derailment. We find here a combination of increased demand for energy with simultaneous lack of oxygen and energy. This situation most likely results from the reduced blood circulation in the area. A vicious cycle develops that ends with the formation of trigger points in the muscle zone with lowered energy supply. Already existing trigger points can likewise be sustained by metabolic derailment.

◾ Muscle Stretching Affects Muscle Metabolism

When contracted sarcomeres (see below) are extended to their greatest length by stretching, this has immediate results for the muscle. First, this reduces the consumption of adenosine triphosphate (ATP) and normalizes metabolism. Second, it decreases muscle tension.

If a metabolic derailment has released substances into the muscle (such as prostaglandin) that can set into motion certain pathomechanisms relevant to trigger points, their concentration declines when the metabolism is returned to normal. It is also suspected that the irritability of the afferent nociceptic nerve fibers is normalized by a balanced metabolism.

◾ The Hypertonic Palpable Muscle Spindle

The hypertonic palpable muscle spindle is a rope-like muscle segment of 1–4 mm thickness surrounding the trigger point, which is noted during palpation because of its greater tightness compared with the surrounding muscle. This spindle stands out due to its hyperesthetic property, to the point of clear painfulness. It is easiest to palpate this hypertonic muscle spindle when its muscle fibers are stretched just to the point where the fibers that are not integrated into the spindle remain relax.

Stretching or strong contraction of the spindle, or pressure on the trigger point within the muscle spindle can cause localized pain and also, after a certain period of latency, referred pain.

Muscle fibers in normal muscles contain sarcomeres that are all the same length. They arrange themselves lengthwise to allow for maximum muscle strength. To achieve this, the actin and myosin filaments must overlap to a certain degree. If they overlap too much or too little, the strength of the muscle is reduced.

Muscle fibers of hypertonic muscle spindles differ histologically: the length of the sarcomeres varies within the spindle. Thus, the sarcomeres around the trigger point are shortened without showing any electromyographic activity—they are **contracted**. Compensating for this, we find lengthened sarcomeres at the end of the muscle spindle near the musculotendinous junction.

This special property explains why a muscle with a hypertonic palpable muscle spindle exhibits reduced stretchability (contracted sarcomeres) as well as reduced strength (shortened and lengthened sarcomeres—sarcomeres outside the ideal length) (**Figs. 14.2–14.4**).

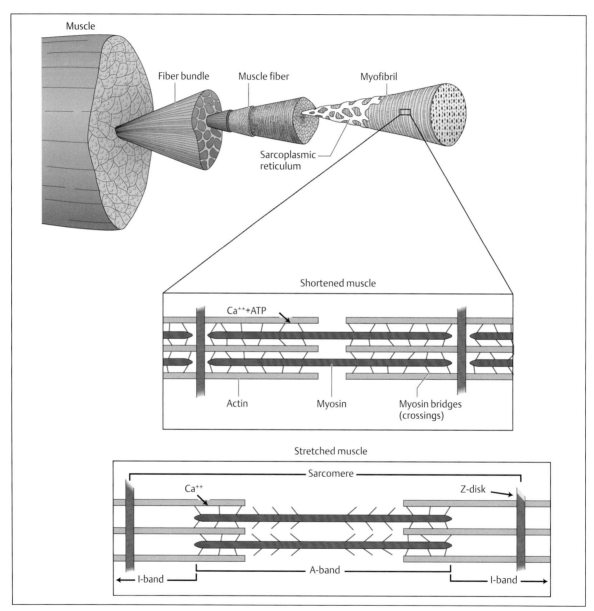

Fig. 14.2 Structure and contractile mechanism in a normal skeletal muscle. The muscle is composed of muscle fiber bundles that consist of striated muscle cells or fibers. An individual fiber generally contains ca. 1000 myofibrils. Every myofibril is surrounded by a tangle with a sack-like structure, the sarcoplasmic reticulum
Enlargements: Adenosine triphosphate (ATP) and free calcium (Ca^{2+}) activate the myosin crossings, as a result of which these pull on the actin filaments. This pull brings the Z-lines closer together and shortens the sarcomeres, the contractile unit by which the muscle is shortened. The segments of actin filaments that do not contain myosin filaments on both sides of a Z-disk form the I-band. The A-band corresponds in length to the myosin filaments. If only an A-, but no I-band exists, a maximal shortening is present

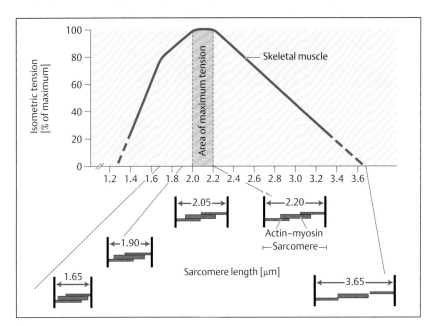

Fig. 14.3   Isometric muscle tone in relation to sarcomere length.

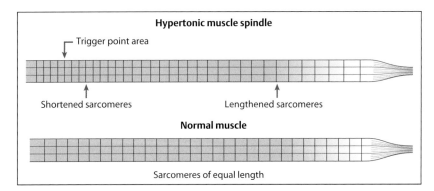

Fig. 14.4   Comparison between sarcomeres of equal length in a normal muscle and the sarcomeres in a muscle with trigger points, which are affected in their length. Shortened sarcomeres in the trigger point region increase tension in the area of the hypertonic muscle spindle and reduce the stretchability of this muscle.

▪ Muscular Weakness and Fast Tiring

Patients with trigger points most likely manifest these symptoms due to reduced circulation and resulting hypoxia in the affected muscle.

15 Diagnosis

The following step-by-step procedure is helpful in the diagnosis of trigger points.

15.1 Detailed Medical History

In order to identify the muscles in which trigger points have formed and that have caused the actual combination of complaints, a precise medical history is needed:

- Did a trauma cause the complaints? Was the onset of pain, for example, preceded by a great effort or did a fall cause the complaints?
- In which position or during which movement did the pain arise for the first time?

- Are there segmental dysfunctions such as joint blockages or prolapsed intervertebral disks that could have facilitated the entire segment?
- Are there any visceral dysfunctions that have hypertonically facilitated the muscles innervated by the same segment in the sense of a viscerosomatic reflex and have encouraged the formation of trigger points?

15.2 Charting Pain Patterns

It can be helpful to chart pain patterns onto a diagram of the body and thereby recognize typical patterns associated with individual muscles. In this context, muscles should be classified according to their historical appearance. It is not uncommon for patterns to overlap. Herein, you should try to answer the following questions:

- Can we create a sequence of occurrence of pain in spite of overlapping patterns? Can we isolate muscle-specific areas?
- In overlapping patterns, are there commonalities, such as identical segmental innervation, which indicates a dysfunction in the context of visceral or structural function?

The pain (as well as increased tension) that a trigger point causes is normally projected and perceived some distance from the localized trigger point. You should also note that the combination of symptoms can vary greatly depending on pain-inducing positions or muscular activity. As a result, complaints can vary considerably within one day as well as from day to day. When pain occurs not only during movements but also when resting, we speak of a greater impairment by trigger points.

In addition to pain, trigger points can also cause incorrect perceptions in surface or depth sensitivity. Even vegetative attendant symptoms in this area can occur, such as increased vasomotoric activity with paleness of the skin during trigger point stimulation, goose bumps, and increased lacrimal and nasal secretion.

15.3 Examining Muscles in Activity

The previously determined muscles are now examined in activity. In this context, we pay attention to pain-triggering positions or movement areas during the entire active movement path. We likewise examine the muscle when passive and active to its position of maximum stretch. We note both the localized pain in the trigger point area as well as the referred pain pattern.

The following results can occur in the presence of trigger points:

- The maximum strength of an affected muscle is reduced in active resistance without indicating atrophy.
- The typical pain patterns can occur or increase when the muscle is worked isometrically or eccentrically.

- Active and passive stretching also triggers referred pain.
- The active and passive stretchability of the muscle is limited.

15.4 Looking for Trigger Points

We now search for trigger points in the specific, previously identified muscles. The examination is performed in neutral position—muscles that are not involved should be neither approximated nor stretched. The finger tip (**Fig. 15.1a–c**) is used to palpate the tissue, perpendicular to the longitudinal axis in superficial muscles (**shallow palpation**). When you encounter a band-like area with obviously elevated tension, you have found the hypertonic muscle spindle with the anticipated trigger point. Within the spindle, you now look for the tenderest spot—the trigger point is identified. Through pressure on this point, you can clearly induce localized and, with sustained pressure, referred pain. The localized pain can arise so strongly, sharply, and spontaneously that patients react with a **"jump" sign**: they twitch, loudly voice pain, or pull the muscle away from the therapist's reach.

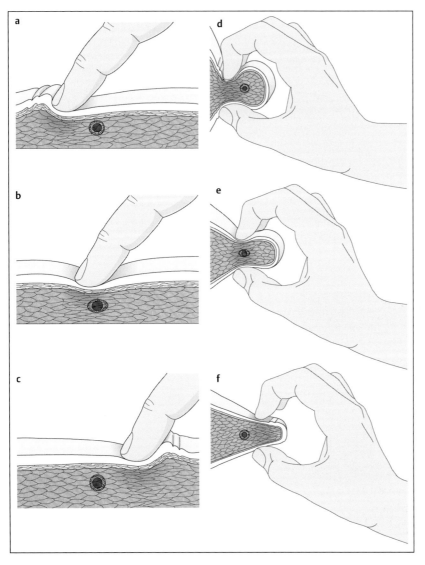

Fig. 15.1a–f **a–c** Cross-section that shows the two-dimensional palpation of a tensed muscle fiber bundle (*black ring*) and its trigger point. Two-dimensional palpation is used with muscles that are only accessible from one side, such as the infraspinatus. **a** At the beginning of palpation, the skin is pushed away. **b** The finger tip glides over the muscle fiber; a tensed fiber bundle can be recognized from its rope-like texture. **c** The skin is lastly pushed to the other side. The same movement is called fast palpation when it is performed more quickly. **d–f** Cross-section illustrating pinching grip palpation of a tensed muscle fiber bundle (*black ring*) at the trigger point. Pinching grip palpation is suited for muscles that can be gripped with the fingers. This applies, for example, to the sternocleidomastoid (SCM) muscles, the pectoralis major, and the latissimus dorsi. **d** Muscle fibers in the pinching grip between thumb and fingers. **e** The tightness of the tensed fiber bundle is clearly detectable when it is rolled around between the fingers. By changing the angle of the finger end joints, a rocking movement is created that allows for better perception of details. **f** The palpable edge of the tensed fiber bundle clearly stands out when it escapes between the finger tips. Often, a local twitch reaction occurs simultaneously

In deeper-lying muscles, identifying the hypertonic muscle spindle can be complicated or made impossible by the over-laying structures. Here, we apply direct **pressure palpation** in the deep tissue to find trigger points.

In the case of muscles that can be grasped between two fingers (such as the trapezius), the **pinching grip** can be useful (**Fig. 15.1d–f**): a section of the muscle belly is rolled back and forth between thumb and index finger to search for the hypertonic muscle spindle. Within the spindle, the same grip is used to find the trigger point.

When palpating a muscle spindle in the vicinity of a trigger point or when directly palpating a trigger point (**Fig. 15.2a**), we can often observe a temporary contraction of the muscle fibers within the muscle spindle. The therapist perceives such a muscle reaction clearly as a visible or palpable twitch (**Fig. 15.2b**). This type of locally limited muscle contraction is par-

ticularly pronounced when palpating across the longitudinal axis of the spindle. Here, the therapist lets the spindle snap back like a guitar string after having stretched it crosswise—as if plucking the guitar string. This **localized twitch reaction** is a characteristic of trigger points.

To determine the location of a trigger point with ultimate certainty, palpation is repeated: an active trigger point presents with reproducible results.

> Pain that originates in the muscles has to be distinguished from neurological, rheumatic, tumorous, psychogenic, inflammatory, and vascular pain.
> Muscle-induced pain comes and goes typically with the activation of the affected muscle by moving or assuming straining positions.

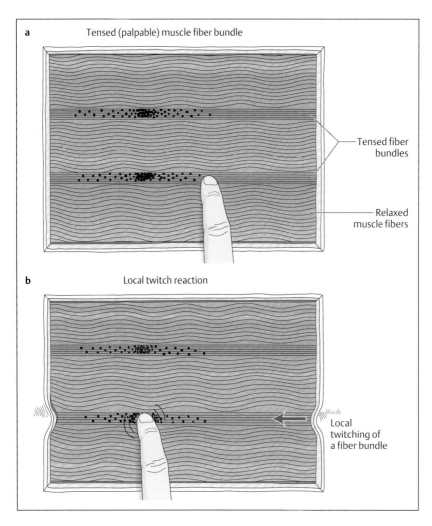

a Tensed (palpable) muscle fiber bundle

Tensed fiber bundles

Relaxed muscle fibers

b Local twitch reaction

Local twitching of a fiber bundle

Fig. 15.2a, b Illustration of a tensed fiber bundle, myofascial trigger points, and a local twitch reaction in a cross-section through the muscle. **a** Palpation of a tensed fiber bundle (*straight lines*) surrounded by slack, relaxed muscle fibers (*wavy lines*). The density of dots reflects the degree of pressure sensitivity in the tensed fiber bundle. The trigger point is the most pressure-sensitive place in the fiber bundle. **b** By rolling the fiber bundle quickly below the finger tip at the location of the trigger point (fast palpation), a local twitch reaction is often caused, which manifests most clearly as the main movement between the trigger point and the attachment of the muscle fibers.

16 Trigger Point Therapy

Besides the different techniques used to treat trigger points, two things are important in therapy:

1. Factors that sustain trigger points will cause prompt and regular reactivation of the trigger points and therefore, of the related complaints in spite of good immediate treatment results. The elimination of these factors is therefore at least as important as the treatment of the muscle.

2. Patients should be involved in the treatment. By this we mean developing sensitivity to straining positions and movements as much as following an individual program of stretching the affected muscles, or whole muscle groups.

16.1 Stretch-and-Spray Technique

This technique aims to deactivate the trigger point by stretching the muscle to its fullest extent without causing reflexive countertension or noteworthy pain.

▪ Applying Cooling Spray

The cooling spray is applied in parallel lines to the skin where the concerned muscle projects to the surface of the body. It must not cause freezing. The spray should merely cause an irritation in the skin for the purpose of creating a "distracting" afferent stimulus that will block the reflexive hypertonicity/spasm in the concerned muscle on the level of the spinal cord.

The spray is applied with a speed of 10 cm/second throughout the entire length of the muscle from a distance of ca. 45 cm and at a 30° angle to the surface. The zone of the referred pain is also included. In the extremities, we work from proximal to distal; at the trunk, from cranial to caudal.

▪ Passive Stretch

After the first two to three applications of spray, we begin by passively stretching the muscle. Slowly, with attention to the prevailing tension barrier, the muscle is extended to its greatest length. We continue to spray uninterruptedly during the stretch stage.

The spray causes a reflexive decrease in tone, as a result of which the stretch can be performed easily without pain. To further support the reflexive relaxation, you can let the patient exhale slowly during the stretch phase and gaze downward.

▪ Active Stretch

The passive range of motion should be exercised actively after the stretch-and-spray. **It is important to emphasize once more: the spraying is a diversion tactic on the level of the spinal cord; the stretch is the treatment**.

16.2   Postisometric Relaxation/Muscle Energy Technique/ Myofascial Release

The muscle is moved into a stretched position to the point where tension prevents further stretching.

The patient is asked to tense against the resistance of the therapist. The therapist gives three-dimensional resistance (ca. 25% of the maximum force) in the direction of the shortening of the muscle without allowing movement (isometric tension). This resistance is sustained for 3–7 seconds.

The patient should relax, and the therapist guides the muscle passively further into extension up to the new tension barrier. Then the procedure is repeated.

After normal muscle length is reached, the new range of motion is exercised actively.

This technique can be increased in effectiveness as well in the relaxation stage by exhaling slowly and looking down.

16.3   Ischemic Compression/Manual Inhibition

Using this technique, the trigger point is treated with manual pressure. The resulting pain must be tolerable and serves as control. When the pain has disappeared after a while (15 seconds to 1 minute), the pressure is increased up to the next pain threshold and the compression is repeated until the trigger point does not hurt any more. The newly gained range of motion is exercised actively.

16.4   Deep Friction Massage

The hypertonic muscle strand with the trigger point is stretched perpendicularly by hand. It is worked along the entire band with constant speed. This technique is painful at first, but the pain must be tolerable to the patient. The stretching is continued until the pain has disappeared (2–3 minutes). Then the newly gained range of motion is exercised actively with the patient.

17 Trigger Point–Sustaining Factors

Factors that sustain trigger points can mean that the performed treatment leads only temporarily to freedom from complaints. Permanent absence of pain is only obtained when these factors are recognized and eliminated. For example, a trigger point can have formed in a muscle as a result of a fall or temporary overexertion. If this trigger point is eliminated soon after the occurrence of the trauma, the body is quickly returned to health. Such treatment successes are the rule in competitive sports because professional athletes undergo constant therapeutic control.

If treatment does not occur immediately after the trauma, the body has time to develop relief positions and evasive movements that protect the injured muscle from further overload. These evasive mechanisms can in turn cause excessive strain in other ligaments, joints, and so on, and trigger new complaints. The original trauma moves to the background and the weakest link in the chain of relief comes to the fore. If the original trigger point was detected in a clinical examination and treated without considering the relief mechanisms that developed later, treatment success will have been neither permanent nor satisfying.

A list of trigger point-sustaining factors follows, without any claims to completeness:

Mechanical Factors

- Leg length differences
- Malpositions in sitting or standing (e.g., double shear forces)
- Spinal column distortions
- Torticollis
- Winged scapula
- Pelvic obliquity (iliac or sacral dysfunctions)
- Coccyx malpositions
- Arm length differences

Systemic Factors

By systemic factors, we mean anything that can negatively affect the energy balance in the muscle. A reduced supply of energy in the muscle supports the formation and preservation of trigger points. Here is a short list of possible systemic factors:
- Lack of vitamin B
- Electrolyte disturbances (e.g., calcium, copper, magnesium, iron)
- Gout
- Anemia
- Hypoglycemia
- Chronic infections
- Weak immune defense
- Psychological stress

18 The Facilitated Segment

The innervation of a spinal cord segment is multi-faceted. The somatic and autonomous nervous systems originate here. On the one hand, the afferent neural fibers run from the posterior horn into the spinal cord; on the other, the efferences leave the segment via the anterior horn. In between, we find a large number of synapses of these two nerve types in the spinal cord itself. By transmitting afferent impulses onto interneurons, diverse modulations become possible for the original neural impulse. Stimuli can be intensified, but they can also be weakened. The mechanisms that cause this phenomenon are partly located at the segmental level, but striking or inhibiting influences from cranial centers, such as via the extrapyramidal system, also have an effect.

If we now consider the afferences on their own, we can divide the spinal cord segment into different sections. We find afferent nerves from the **sclerotome**. By this, we mean not only the neural supply in the bones, but also in the joints (including cartilage), joint capsules, fasciae, synovium, and ligaments. The perception of depth sensitivity and pain is the task of these sclerotome neurons.

Equally innervated segmentally is the musculature—the **myotome**. Muscles also supply information about depth sensitivity and pain through their associated fiber and tendon sensors.

A skin area that is innervated exclusively by a spinal cord segment is the **dermatome**. Surface sensitivity is perceived through afference here.

The last innervated area of a segment is the **viscerotome**. Afferent information about pain or generally harmful agencies is conducted to the spinal cord.

What applies for the afferences also holds true for the efferences. Every area of innervation is also approached efferently from the spinal cord: In this way, the fasciae or muscles in the skin, internal organs, or skeletal muscles are supplied motorically.

All this is, so to speak, the hardware of the segment. The software is what we refer to as a "**facilitated segment.**" Afferent stimuli are largely processed and modulated at the level of the spinal cord, and then answered as efferent impulse. In some cases, this processing can include all the innervated areas of the segment, and the response can be equally multi-leveled.

Example: A person suffers from duodenal ulcer. The information about the damage to the mucus is transmitted to the spinal cord through visceral afferences. A response to this information will now challenge the entire segment. On the one hand, the viscerotome

can react: the smooth muscles become hypertonic—a spasm in the intestinal wall arises. Through spinal cord synapses we could also expect a response in the dermatome: segmental areas of the abdominal wall can manifest hyperesthesia, circulatory changes (paleness or redness), or pilomotoric activity. The sclerotome reacts with fascial contraction in the damaged area so that the inflamed section of the intestines is immobilized. Alternately, segmental joint blockages develop in the physiological motion pattern. And lastly, we can see the formation of trigger points in the myotome, that is, in the abdominal musculature. This complex segmental reaction serves the cause of regeneration, of the body's self-healing: all sections of the body work to remove the ulcer from the duodenum.

If healing is successful, two areas of reaction in particular may continue their immobilizing efforts, in spite of the fact that it is no longer necessary: the fasciae and the muscles. As far as the muscles are concerned, we can say that the trigger point activity should be removed by the therapy because otherwise a limitation of movement persists, which can in turn become the source for new pathologies. The same applies to the fascial tension.

For each muscle, this book lists the associated organs because the chain of reaction can also proceed in the reverse order:
When you find trigger points in a muscle, you should also observe the segmentally matched organs, test for a potential dysfunction, and treat them. If you only remove the trigger point and overlook a visceral dysfunction, this will either result in no relief from complaints at all in the musculature, or in later relapses.

The "facilitated segment" continually challenges the therapist to abandon one-dimensional thinking, to employ neuroanatomy, and to place the symptoms in the larger segmental context. Therapists should not limit themselves to treating only a trigger point to remove, for example, a painful shoulder movement. The complexity of our body deserves more. If therapists commit to this, they will obtain much better and longer-lasting therapeutic results.

19 The Trigger Points

19.1 Muscles of Head and Neck Pain

With active trigger points (TP), the muscles in this section lead to pain in the head and neck region, which could be misinterpreted as one of the following:
• Migraine
• Arthrosis of the temporomandibular joint

• Sinusitis
• Pharyngitis
• Laryngitis
• Dental disease
• Trigeminal neuralgia etc.

▪ Trapezius Muscle (Figs. 19.1, 19.2, 19.3, 19.4)

Origin

• Middle third of the superior nuchal line
• Nuchal ligaments
• Spinous processes and supraspinous ligament up to T12.

Insertion

• Outer third of the back border of the clavicle
• Medial section of the acromion
• Upper border of the spine of the scapula

Action

• Outward rotation in the shoulder joint
• Lifting the scapula
• Retracting the scapula to the spinal column
• In cases with fixed scapula: extension and lateral flexion of the thoracic spinal column (TSC)

Innervation

• Accessorius nerve
• Proprioceptive fibers from C3/C4

Trigger Point Location

Trigger points of the trapezius are found throughout the entire muscle:

TP1 In the free border of the descending part palpable as hypertonic bands

TP2 Posterior of TP1 and above the scapular spine—around the center of the spine

TP3 In the region of the lateral rim of the descending part, near the medial border of the scapula

TP4 In the ascending part directly below the scapular spine, near the medial border of the scapula

TP5 In the horizontal part ca. 1 cm medial of the insertion of the levator scapula muscle on the scapula

TP6 In the supraspinatous fossa of the scapula, near the acromion

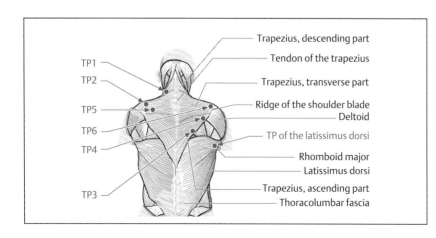

Fig. 19.1

TP1
TP2
TP5
TP6
TP4
TP3

Trapezius, descending part
Tendon of the trapezius
Trapezius, transverse part
Ridge of the shoulder blade
Deltoid
TP of the latissimus dorsi
Rhomboid major
Latissimus dorsi
Trapezius, ascending part
Thoracolumbar fascia

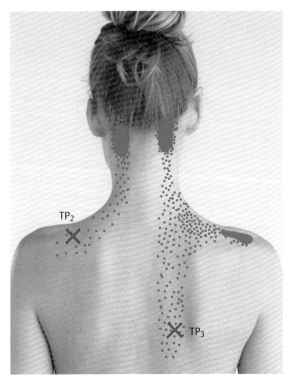

Fig. 19.2

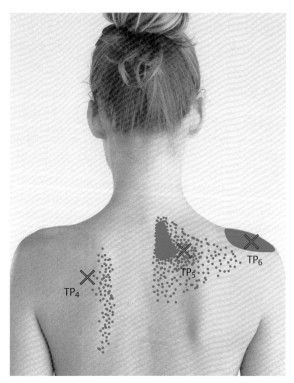

Fig. 19.3

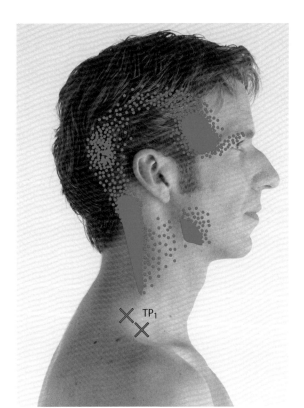

Fig. 19.4

Referred Pain

TP1 Posterolateral in the throat and neck region up to the mastoid process
Lateral at the head—especially in the temple region and eye socket, temporomandibular joint

TP2 Mastoid process and upper cervical spinal column (CSC) (posterolateral)

TP3 Mastoid process and upper CSC (posterolateral) and in the area of the acromion

TP4 Along the medial border of the scapula

TP5 Paravertebral between C7 and TP5

TP6 Roof of the shoulders, acromion

Associated Internal Organs

- Liver
- Gallbladder
- Stomach

▪ Sternocleidomastoid Muscle (Figs. 19.5, 19.6, 19.7)

Origin

- Ventrocranial at the manubrium
- Upper rim of the medial third of the clavicle

Insertion

- Outside of the mastoid process
- Lateral half of the superior nuchal line

Action

- Ipsilateral lateral flexion and contralateral rotation of the CSC
- Double-sided contraction: extension of the CSC with ventral translation

Innervation

- Accessorius nerve

Trigger Point Location

Trigger points are found in the sternal and clavicular section throughout the entire length of the muscle.

Referred Pain

Trigger points of the sternocleidomastoid muscle (SCM) lead to facial pain, which can easily be mistaken for trigeminal neuralgia.

Trigger Points in the Sternal Section

- Manubrium
- Supraorbital and in the orbita
- Cheek
- Outer auditory canal
- Temporomandibular joint region
- Pharynx and tongue
- Occiput, posterior to the mastoid process

Trigger Points in the Clavicular Section

- Forehead, potentially also on both sides
- Outer auditory canal
- Immediately behind the ear

Associated Internal Organs

- Liver
- Gallbladder
- Stomach

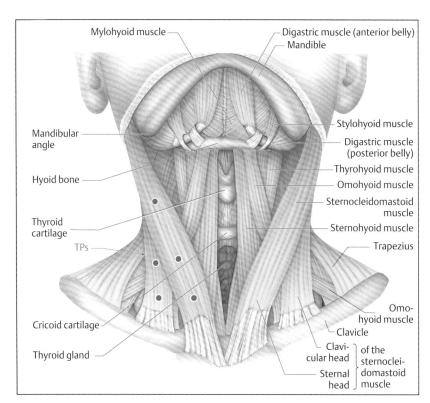

Fig. 19.5

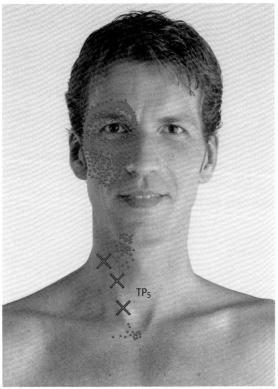

Fig. 19.6

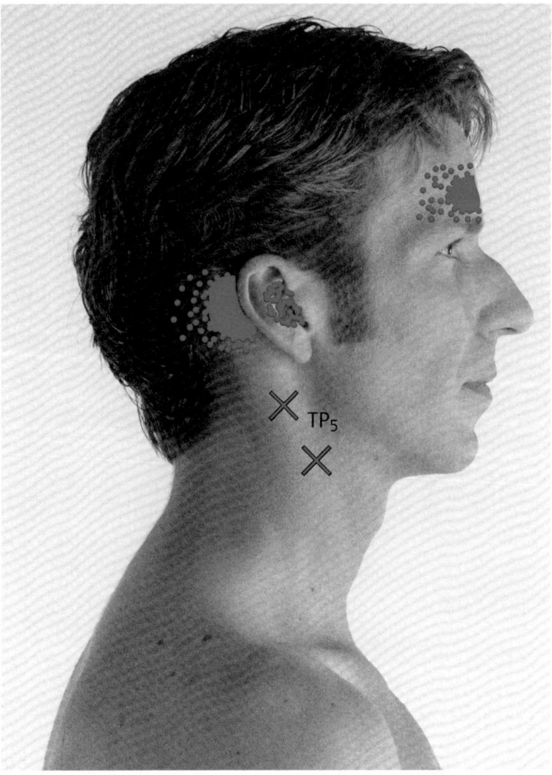

Fig. 19.7

■ Masseter Muscle (Figs. 19.8, 19.9)

Origin

- Frontal two-thirds of the zygomatic arch
- Zygomatic process of the maxilla

Insertion

- Outside of the mandibular joint
- Lower section of the mandibular branch

Action

- Lifting the lower jaw (closing the mouth)

Innervation

Mandibular nerve (trigeminal nerve)

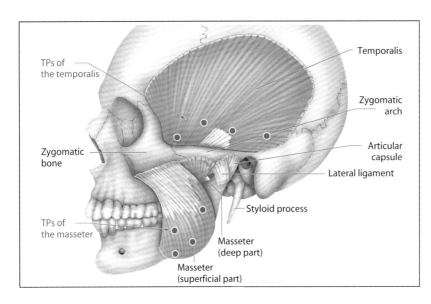

Fig. 19.8

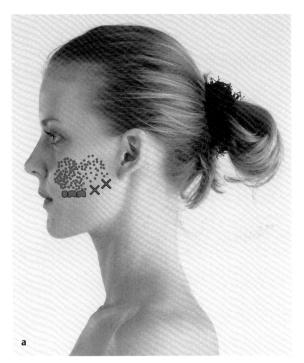

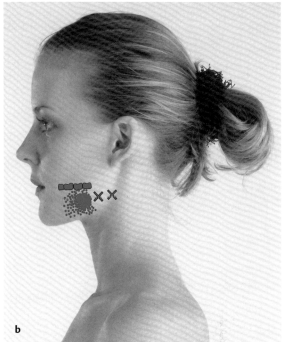

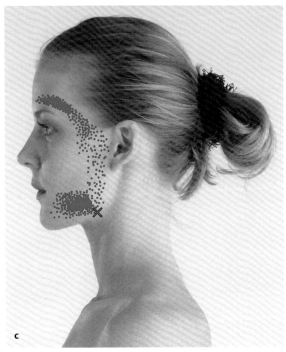

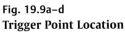

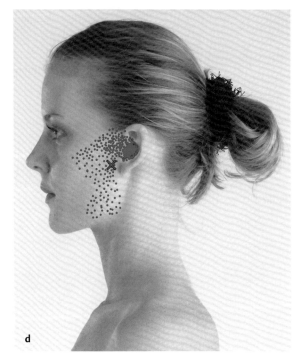

Fig. 19.9a–d
Trigger Point Location

Trigger points are found distributed throughout the entire muscle.

Referred Pain

- Maxilla and upper molars
- Mandible and lower molars
- From the temple to above the eyebrows

- Temporomandibular joint
- Outer auditory canal

Sometimes trigger points cause tinnitus in the masseter.

Associated Internal Organs

None

■ Temporalis Muscle (Fig. 19.10a–d)

Origin

Temporal bone between the inferior temporal line and the infratemporal crest

Insertion

Medial and ventral section of the coronoid process of the mandible

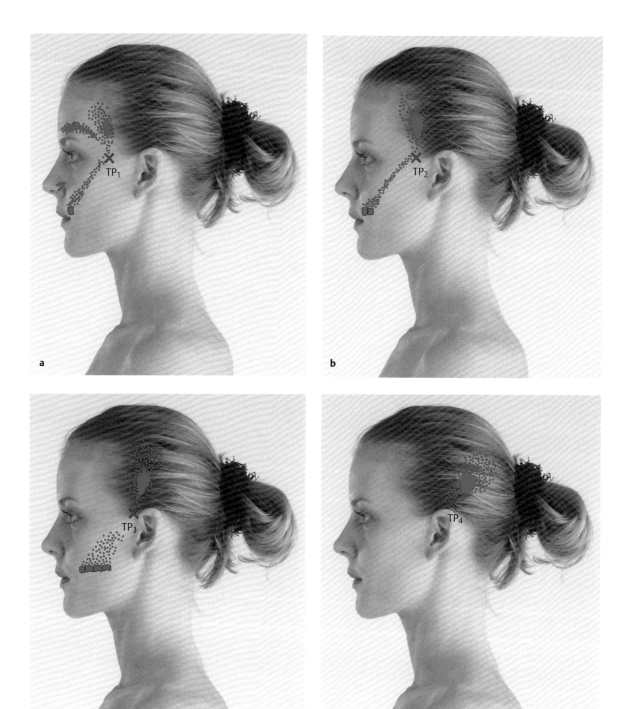

Fig. 19.10a–d

Action

Raising and guiding back the lower jaw

Innervation

Mandibular nerve (trigeminal nerve)

Trigger Point Location

TP1–3   Found above the zygomatic process.
TP4   Above the ear (see also **Fig. 19.8**)

Referred Pain

- From the temple to parietal
- Above the eyebrow
- Upper row of teeth
- Behind the eye

Associated Internal Organs

None

▪ Lateral Pterygoid Muscle (Figs. 19.11, 19.12)

Origin

- Underside of the greater wing of the sphenoid bone
- Outside of the lateral pterygoid plate

Insertion

- Pterygoid bone below the condyloid process of the mandible
- Articular disk of the temporomandibular joint

Action

Opening the mouth (pulling the lower jaw forward, which also pulls the disk forward)

Innervation

Lateral pterygoid nerve from the mandibular nerve (trigeminal nerve)

Trigger Point Location

The trigger points of this short muscle are found by intraoral palpation roughly in the middle of the muscle belly.

Referred Pain

- Temporomandibular joint
- Maxilla

Associated Internal Organs

None

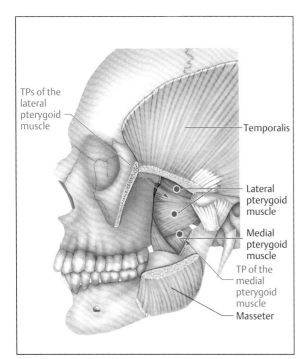

Fig. 19.11

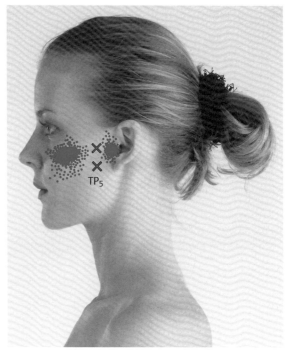

Fig. 19.12

■ Medial Pterygoid Muscle (Fig. 19.13)

Origin

- Inside the lateral pterygoid plate
- Pterygoid bone
- Maxillary tuberosity
- Pyramidal process of the palatine bone

Insertion

Inside the mandibular joint

Action

Moving the lower jaw forward, upward, and lateral (chewing)

Innervation

Medial pterygoid nerve from the mandibular nerve (trigeminal nerve)

Trigger Point Location

The trigger points of this short muscle are found by intraoral palpation roughly in the middle of the muscle belly (see also **Fig. 19.11**, page 131).

Referred Pain

- Tongue
- Pharynx
- Larynx
- Temporomandibular joint

Associated Internal Organs

None

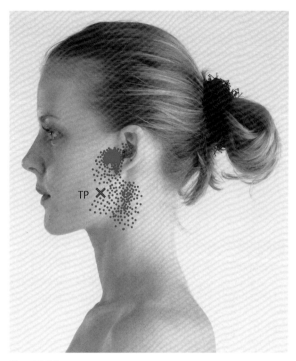

Fig. 19.13

■ Digastric Muscle (Figs. 19.14, 19.15)

Origin

- Ventral head: digastric fossa on the backside of the symphysis menti
- Dorsal head: mastoid notch on the mastoid process

Insertion

On the intermediate tendon that inserts laterally on the hyoid bone

Action

- Lifting the hyoid bone
- Pulling the mandible forward
- Supports the process of swallowing

Innervation

- Ventral head: mandibular nerve (trigeminal nerve)
- Dorsal head: facial nerve

Trigger Point Location

The trigger points are palpated along the course of the muscle as hypersensitive points medial to the SCM muscle.

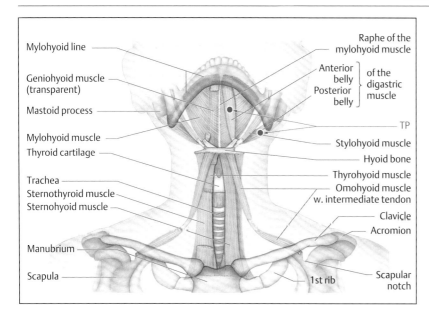

Fig. 19.14

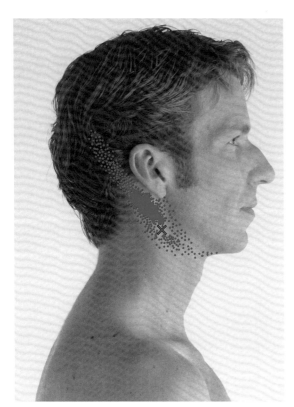

Fig. 19.15

Referred Pain

- Dorsal head:
  - into the upper region of the SCM muscle
  - occiput
  - neck region, near the mandible
- Ventral head: lower incisors and the mandibles underneath

Associated Internal Organs

None

▪ Orbicularis Oculi, Zygomaticus Major, and Platysma Muscles (Fig. 19.16)

Orbicularis Oculi

Origin

Medial orbita rim, wall of the lacrimal sac

Insertion

Palpebral ligament

Action

Closing the eyelids, supporting tearing

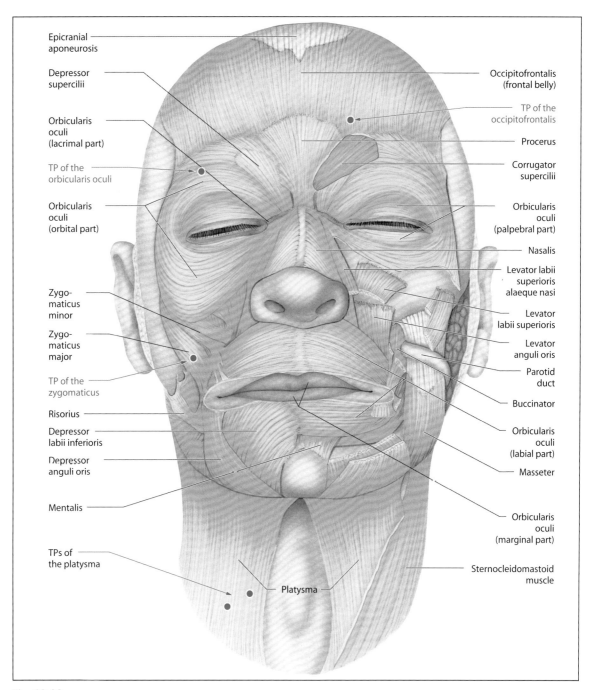

Fig. 19.16

Zygomaticus Major Muscle

Origin

Foreside of the zygomatic bone

Insertion

Lateral to the corner of the mouth

Action

Pulling the corners of the mouth backward and up-ward

Platysma Muscle

Origin

Skin in the lower neck region and upper exterior thorax region

Insertion

Lower edge of the mandible, skin in the lower facial region, corner of the mouth

Action

Pulling the skin of the lower face and mouth regions and the lower jaw downward

Innervation

Facial nerve

Trigger Point Location

Orbicularis Oculi

Above the eyelid, immediately below the eyebrow

Zygomaticus Major

In the area of the muscle near the insertion—craniolateral to the corner of the mouth

Platysma

Ca. 2 cm above the clavicle on the intersection with the SCM muscle

Referred Pain

Orbicularis Oculi

- Bridge of the nose
- Upper lip

Zygomaticus Major

Originating from the trigger point, lateral to the nose and medial to the eyes, to the forehead (center)

Platysma

- Mandible
- Cheek
- Chin

Associated Internal Organs

None

▪ Occipitofrontalis Muscle (Figs. 19.17, 19.18)

Origin

- Superior nuchal line, mastoid process
- Referring to the fibers of the upper facial muscles

Insertion

Epicranial aponeurosis

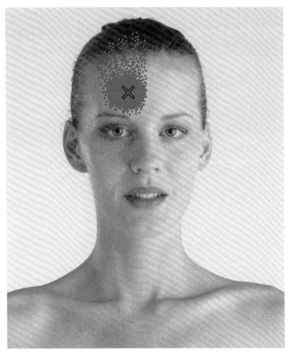

Fig. 19.17

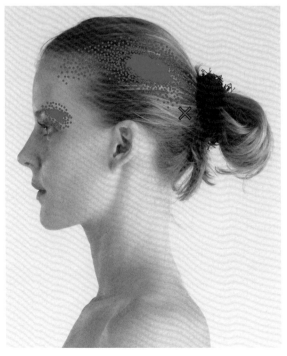

Fig. 19.18

Action

- Stabilizing the epicranial aponeurosis
- Wrinkling the forehead

Innervation

Facial nerve

Trigger Point Location

- Frontal: above the medial end of the eyebrow

- Occipital: above the superior nuchal line and ca. 4 cm lateral to the center line (see also **Fig. 19.16**, p. 134)

Referred Pain

This originates from the orbita, across the ipsilateral half of the skull along the course of the muscle.

Associated Internal Organs

None

■ Splenius Capitis and Cervicis Muscles (Figs. 19.19, 19.20)

Origin

- Splenius capitis: nuchal line and spinous processes and supraspinous ligaments T1–T3

- Splenius cervicis: spinous processes and supraspinous ligaments T3–T6

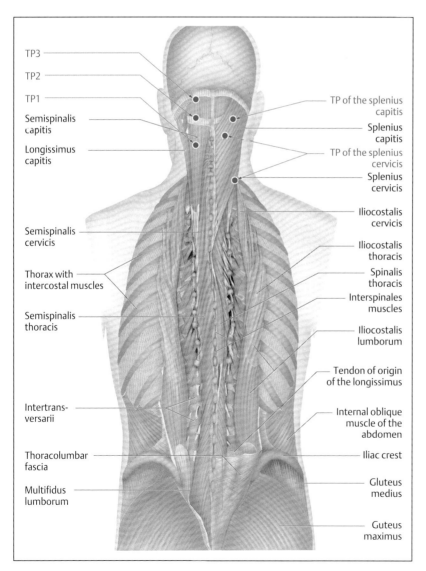

Fig. 19.19

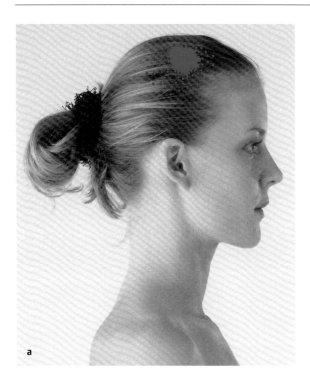

Fig. 19.20a–c

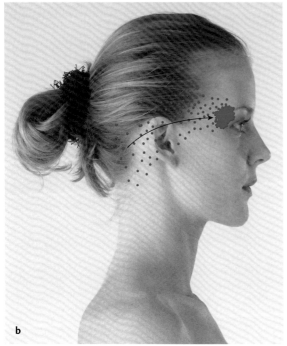

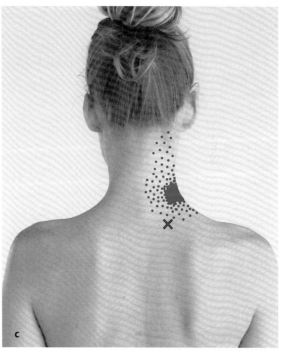

Insertion

- Splenius capitis: between the superior and inferior nuchal ligaments (lateral to the occiput)
- Splenius cervicis: posterior tubercle C1–C3

Action

Extension and ipsilateral rotation of the CSC

Innervation

- Splenius capitis: spinal nerves C3/C4 (dorsal branches)
- Splenius cervicis: spinal nerves C5/C6 (dorsal branches)

Trigger Point Location

- Splenius capitis: in the muscle belly roughly at the height of the spinous process of the axis
- Splenius cervicis: at the height of the transition from the shoulder to the neck and a little further up from there a second trigger point near the muscle insertion at the level of C2/C3

For palpation, slide the palpating finger between the trapezius and levator scapulae.

Referred Pain

- Splenius capitis: into the vertex of the skull—ipsilateral
- Splenius cervicis: through the skull to behind the eye, sometimes also to the occiput, shoulder–neck transition, and ascending ipsilateral up the neck

Associated Internal Organs

- Liver
- Gallbladder

■ Semispinalis Capitis and Cervicis Muscles, Multifidus Muscles (Transversospinalis) (Figs. 19.21, 19.22)

Origin

- Semispinalis: transverse processes
- Multifidus: lamina

Insertion

- Semispinalis: spinous processes (ca. six vertebrae cranial to the origin)
- Multifidus: spinous processes (ca. two to three vertebrae cranial to the origin)

These muscles run approximately between the T6 and the superior/inferior nuchal line.

Action

Extension and lateral flexion ipsilateral to the spinal column

Innervation

Dorsal branches of the segmental spinal nerve

Trigger Point Location

TP1   At the base of the neck at the level of C4/C5
TP2   2–4 cm below the occiput
TP3   Immediately below the superior nuchal line (see also **Fig. 19.19**)

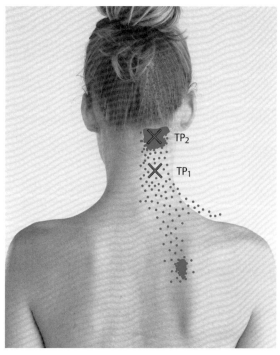

Fig. 19.21

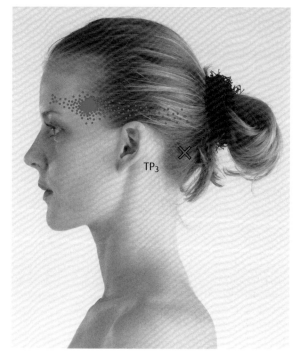

Fig. 19.22

Referred Pain

TP1   Along the neck up into the suboccipital region and also caudally up to the medial border of the scapula

TP2   From the occiput towards the vertex

TP3   Painful band sideways across the skull up to the temple region

Associated Internal Organs

- Heart
- Lung/bronchial tubes

■ Rectus Capitis Posterior Major and Minor Muscles, Obliquus Capitis Inferior and Superior Muscles (Figs. 19.23, 19.24)

Origin

- Rectus capitis posterior major: spinous process C2
- Rectus capitis posterior minor: posterior tubercle of the atlas
- Obliquus capitis inferior: spinous process C2
- Obliquus capitis superior: lateral mass of the atlas

Insertion

- Rectus capitis posterior major: outer half of the inferior nuchal line
- Rectus capitis posterior minor: medial half of the inferior nuchal line
- Obliquus capitis inferior: lateral mass of the atlas
- Obliquus capitis superior: lateral half of the inferior nuchal line

Action

- Rectus capitis posterior major: extension of the head and ipsilateral rotation in the atlantooccipital joint
- Rectus capitis posterior minor: extension of the head
- Obliquus capitis inferior: ipsilateral rotation in the atlantoaxial joint
- Obliquus capitis superior: sideways inclination of the head

Innervation

- Suboccipital nerve (dorsal branch of C1)

Trigger Point Location

In the muscle belly, only general tension is palpable, but not a definable trigger point.

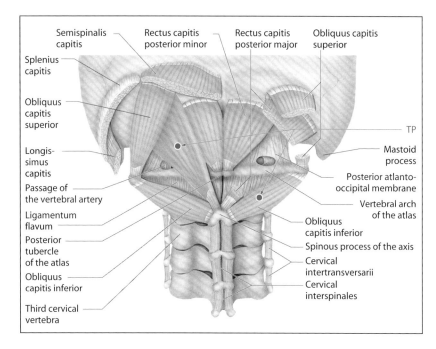

Fig. 19.23

Referred Pain

From the occiput through the temple region up to the orbita and forehead (ipsilateral). The pain is not exactly and clearly localizable.

Associated Internal Organs

None

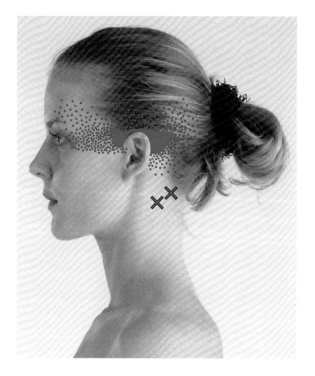

Fig. 19.24

19.2 Muscles of Upper Thorax Pain and Shoulder–Arm Pain

▪ Levator Scapulae Muscle (Figs. 19.25, 19.26)

Origin

Posterior tubercle C1–C4

Insertion

Medial border of the scapula (cranial)

Action

- Rotation of the caudal scapular angle to medial, and elevation of the cranial scapular angle to cranial-medial
- Extension (double-sided contraction) and ipsilateral rotation of the CSC

Innervation

Dorsal scapular nerve (C5) and ventral branches of the spinal nerves C3–C4

Trigger Point Location

TP1 Shoulder-neck transition, palpable when trapezius is displaced to posterior

TP2 Ca. 1.3 cm above the upper scapular angle

Referred Pain

- Transition from the shoulder to the neck
- Medial scapular border
- Dorsal shoulder region

Associated Internal Organs

- Liver
- Gallbladder
- Stomach
- Heart

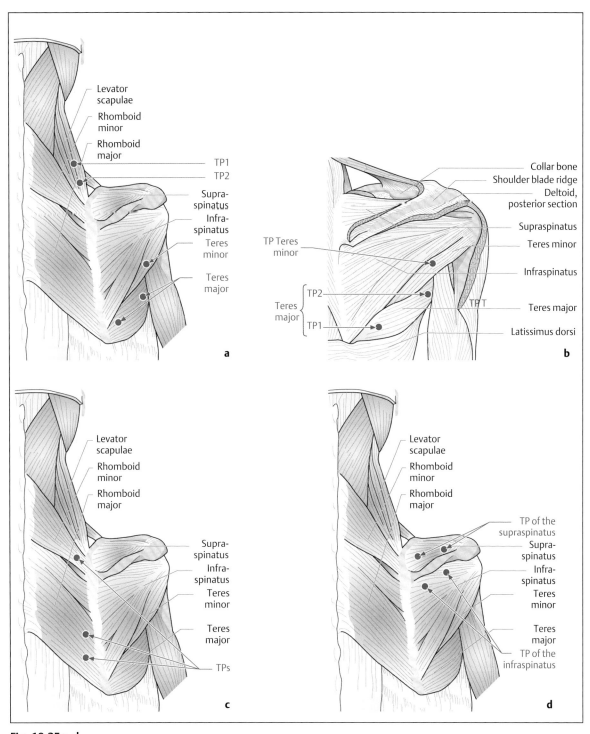

Fig. 19.25a–d

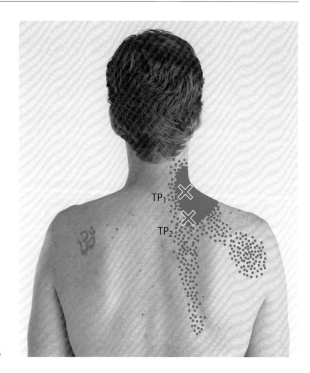

Fig. 19.26

■ Scalene Muscles (Figs. 19.27, 19.28, 19.29)

Origin

- Scalenus anterior: anterior tubercles C3–C6
- Scalenus medius: posterior tubercles C2–C7
- Scalenus posterior: posterior tubercles C4–C6
- Scalenus minimus: anterior tubercle C7

Insertion

- Scalenus anterior: scalene tubercle of the first rib
- Scalenus medius: upper edge of the first rib (near neck of rib)
- Scalenus posterior: lateral posterior outside of the second rib
- Scalenus minimus: suprapleural membrane

Action

- Inhalatory muscles
- Scalenus anterior: additionally supports the lateral flexion of the CSC when the rib is fixed
- Scalenus minimus: tenses the pleural dome

Innervation
Ventral branches of the spinal nerves:
- Scalenus anterior: C5–C6
- Scalenus medius: C3–C8
- Scalenus posterior: C6–C8
- Scalenus minimus: C7

Trigger Point Location

The scalene muscles are found in the fossa supraclavicularis major and are partly compressed against the transverse processes of the cervical vertebrae. The trigger points are distributed in the muscles at varying heights.

Referred Pain

- Chest area
- Radial ventral and dorsal upper arm and forearm

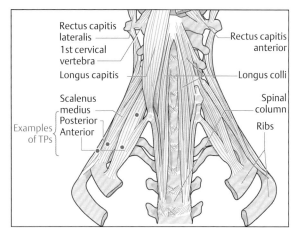

Fig. 19.27

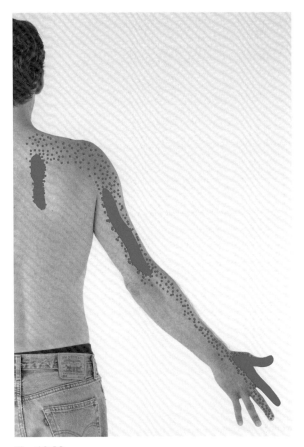

Fig. 19.28

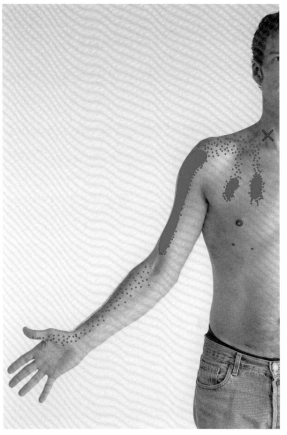

Fig. 19.29

- Thumb and index finger from dorsal (scalenus minimus: entire back of the hand)
- Medial border of the scapula

This referred pain can be confused with the pain pattern of a heart attack!

Associated Internal Organs

See teres major muscle.

■ Supraspinatus Muscle (Figs. 19.30, 19.31)

Origin

- Supraspinous fossa of the scapula
- Spine of the scapula

Insertion

- Greater tubercle of the humerus (proximal facet)
- Shoulder joint capsule

Action

- Abduction of the arm
- Shoulder joint stabilizer

Innervation

Suprascapular nerve (C5–C6)

Trigger Point Location

Both trigger points are easily palpable in the supraspinous fossa of the scapula.

Referred Pain

- Lateral deltoid area
- Lateral epicondyle
- Lateral upper arm and forearm
- Shoulder roof

Associated Internal Organs

See Teres Major Muscle (p. 146).

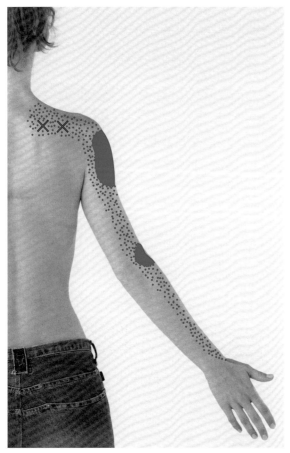

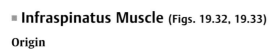

Fig. 19.30

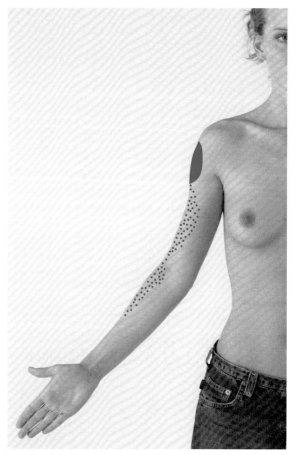

Fig. 19.31

■ Infraspinatus Muscle (Figs. 19.32, 19.33)

Origin

Infraspinous fossa of the scapula

Insertion

• Greater tubercle of the humerus (middle facet)
• Shoulder joint capsule

Action

• Outward rotation of the arm
• Shoulder joint stabilizer

Innervation

Suprascapular nerve (C5–C6)

Trigger Point Location

TP1 is found in the infraspinous fossa immediately below the spine of the scapula near the medial border of the scapula; TP2 somewhat further laterally (see also **Fig. 19.25**).

Referred Pain

• Ventral shoulder area
• Ventrolateral upper arm and forearm
• Radial palm and back of the hand

Associated Internal Organs

See Teres Major Muscle (p. 146).

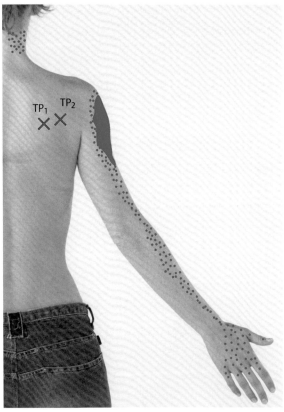

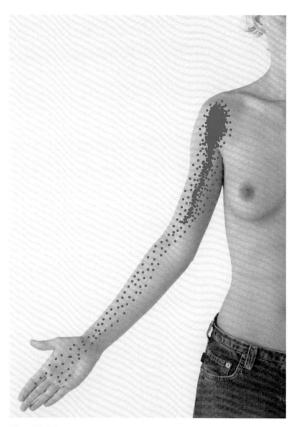

Fig. 19.32

Fig. 19.33

▪ Teres Minor Muscle (Fig. 19.34)

Origin

Lateral border of the scapula (middle third), above the teres major

Insertion

- Greater tubercle of the humerus (lower facet)
- Shoulder joint capsule

Action

- Outward rotation of the arm
- Shoulder joint stabilizer

Innervation

Axillary nerve (C5–C6)

Trigger Point Location

In the lateral of the lateral border of the scapula between the infraspinatus and teres major muscles

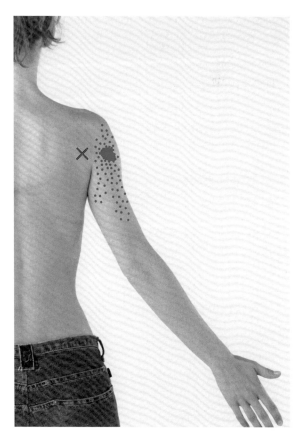

Fig. 19.34

Referred Pain

- Posterior deltoid area, a little above the deltoid insertion
- Posterior upper arm

Associated Internal Organs

See teres major muscle below.

■ Teres Major Muscle (Fig. 19.35)

Origin

- Distal third of the lateral border of the scapula (below the teres minor)
- Inferior angle of the scapula

Insertion

Crest of the lesser tubercle of the humerus

Action

- Inward rotation
- Adduction
- Shoulder joint stabilizer

Innervation

Subscapular nerve (C5–C6)

Trigger Point Location

TP1   In the area of the lower angle of the scapula
TP2   Lateral in the muscle belly in the posterior axillary fold (see also **Fig. 19.25**)

Referred Pain

- Dorsal deltoid area
- Along the long head of the triceps
- Dorsal forearm

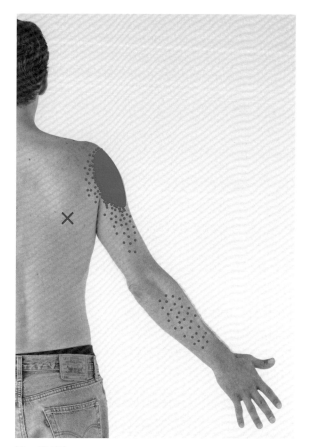

Fig. 19.35

Associated Internal Organs

- The scalene, supraspinatus, infraspinatus, teres major and minor, and deltoid muscles often develop trigger points as a result of slipped cervical disks (C4/C5, C5/C6, C6/C7)
- Heart

■ Latissimus Dorsi Muscle (Fig. 19.36)

Origin

- Spinous processes and supraspinous ligaments of all cervical, lumbar, and sacral vertebrae from T7 downward
- Thoracolumbar fascia
- Iliac crest (rear third)
- Ribs 9–12
- Inferior angle of the scapula

Insertion

Crest of the lesser tubercle of the humerus

Action

- Extension, internal rotation, and adduction of the arm
- Deep inhalation and forced expiration

Innervation

Thoracodorsal nerve (C6–C8)

Trigger Point Location

In the free border of the posterior axillary fold around the height of the middle of the lateral border of the scapula (also see **Fig. 19.1**)

Referred Pain

- Lower angle of the scapula and circular in its vicinity
- Dorsal shoulder area
- Dorsomedial upper arm and forearm inclusive of fingers 4 and 5

Associated Internal Organs

None

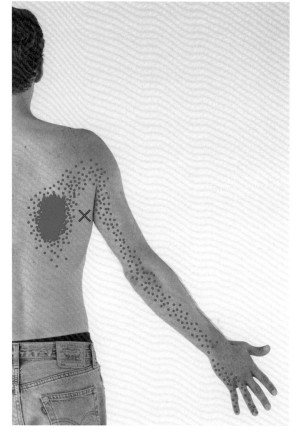

Fig. 19.36

▪ Subscapularis Muscle (Figs. 19.37, 19.38)

Origin

Subscapular fossa

Insertion

- Lesser tubercle of the humerus
- Crest of the lesser tubercle of the humerus (proximal)
- Shoulder joint capsule

Action

- Inward rotation
- Shoulder joint stabilizer

Innervation

Subscapular nerve (C6–C7)

Trigger Point Location

Near the lateral border of the scapula in the subscapular fossa. In addition, you find trigger points in the subscapular fossa further medially in the direction of the upper angle of the scapula.

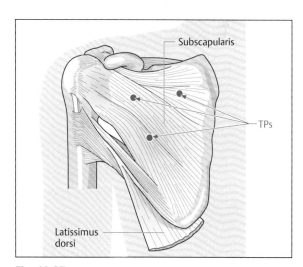

Fig. 19.37

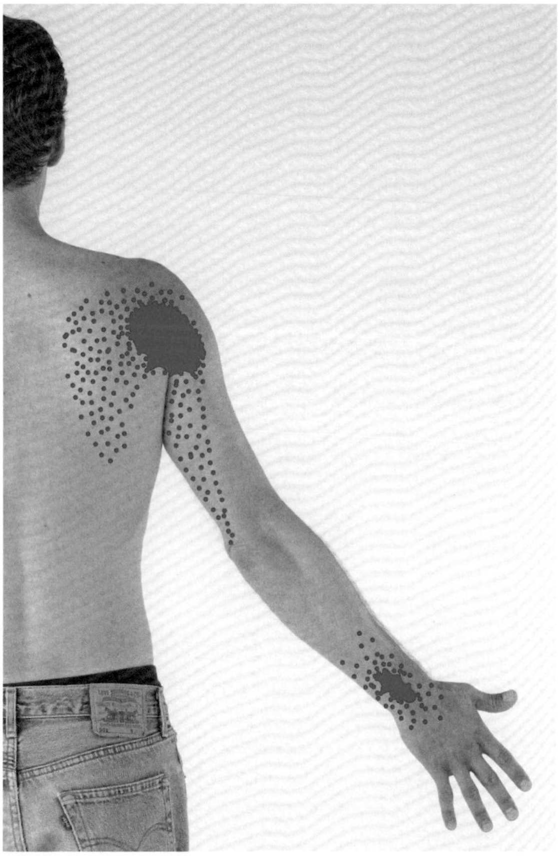

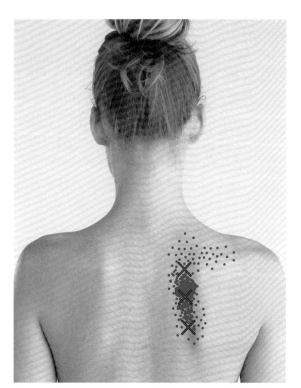

Fig. 19.38

Referred Pain

- Posterior shoulder area
- Entire surface of the scapula
- Dorsal upper arm up to the elbow
- Hand joint (dorsal and palmar)

Associated Internal Organs

None

▪ Rhomboid Muscle (Fig. 19.39)

Origin

- Nuchal ligament
- Spinous processes and supraspinous ligaments C7–T5

Insertion

Medial border of the scapula

Action

Retraction of the scapula

Innervation

Dorsal scapular nerve (C5)

Trigger Point Location

Along and near the medial border of the scapula (see also **Fig. 19.25**)

Fig. 19.39

Referred Pain

• Along the medial border of the scapula between the scapula and the paravertebral musculature
• Supraspinous fossa of the scapula

Associated Internal Organs

Heart

■ Deltoid Muscle (Figs. 19.40, 19.41, 19.42)

Origin

• Clavicle (lateral third)
• Acromion
• Spine of the scapula

Insertion

Deltoid tuberosity

Action

• Abduction of the arm
• Ventral section: flexion, internal rotation
• Dorsal section: extension, external rotation

Innervation

Axillary nerve (C5–C6)

Trigger Point Location

• Ventral trigger points: in the upper third of the muscle belly in front of the glenohumeral joint and in the vicinity of its anterior border
• Dorsal trigger points: along the posterior edge of the muscle belly in its lower half

Referred Pain

• Ventral trigger points: anterior and lateral deltoid area and upper arm
• Dorsal trigger points: posterior and lateral deltoid area and upper arm

Associated Internal Organs

See Teres Major Muscle (p. 146).

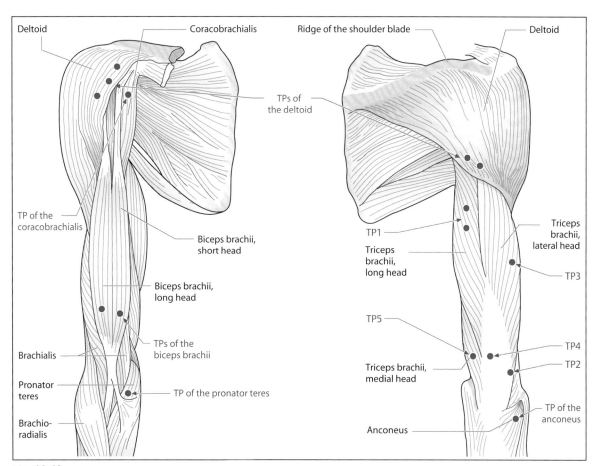

Fig. 19.40

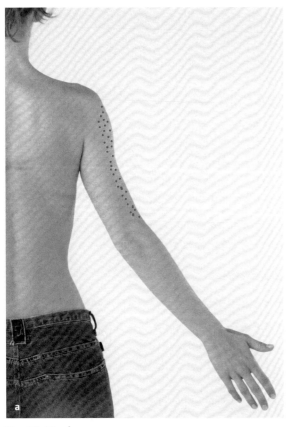
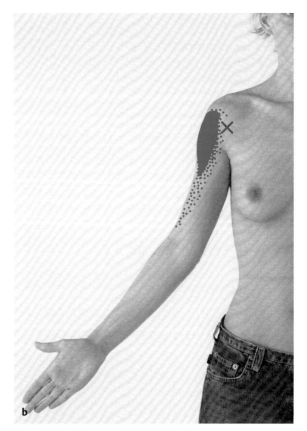

Fig. 19.41a, b

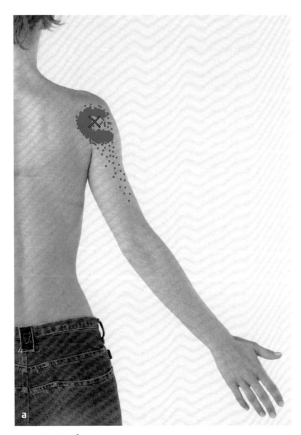
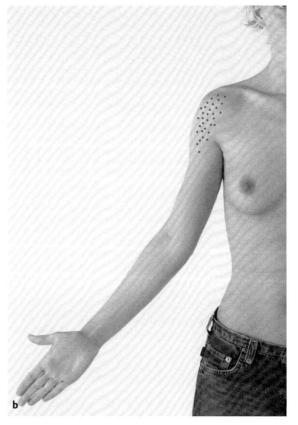

Fig. 19.42a, b

▪ Coracobrachialis Muscle (Fig. 19.43)

Origin

Coracoid process of the scapula

Insertion

Medial side of the humerus (proximal half)

Action

Flexion, adduction of the arm

Innervation

Musculocutaneous nerve (C5–C7)

Trigger Point Location

Palpate in the armpit between the deltoid and pectoralis major and press the muscle in its cranial section against the humerus.

Referred Pain

- Anterior aspect of the deltoid
- In a continuous line on parts of the upper arm, forearm, and back of the hand

Associated Internal Organs

None

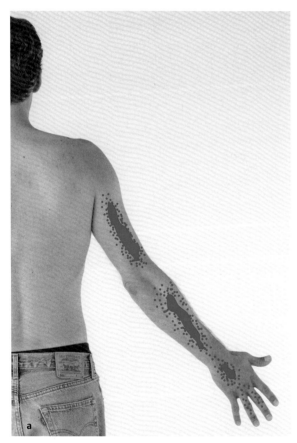 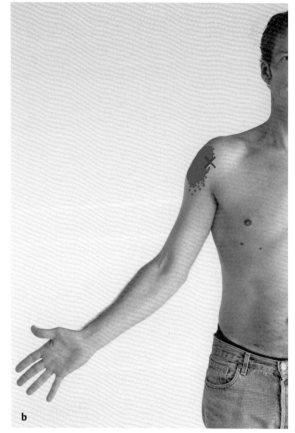

Fig. 19.43a, b

■ Biceps Brachii Muscle (Fig. 19.44)

Origin

- Long head: supraglenoid tubercle of the scapula
- Short head: coracoid process of the scapula

Insertion

- Radial tuberosity
- Bicipital aponeurosis

Action

- Flexion of the arm
- Flexion of the elbow
- Supination of the forearm

Innervation

Musculocutaneous nerve (C5–C6)

Trigger Point Location

In the distal third of the muscle (see **Fig. 19.40**)

Referred Pain

- Ventral deltoid area
- Ventral upper arm in the course of the muscle
- Inner side of the elbow joint
- Suprascapular region

Associated Internal Organs

None

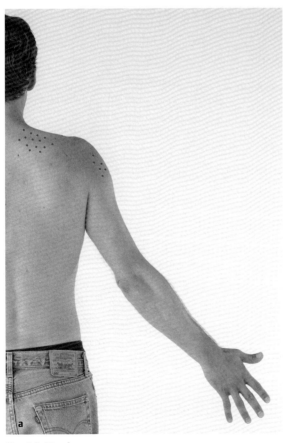
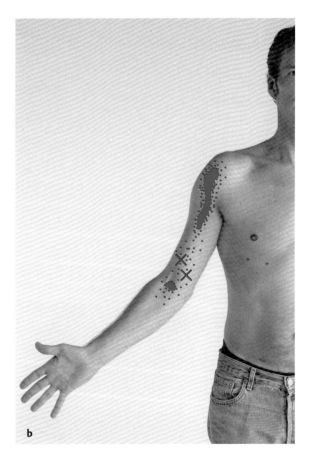

Fig. 19.44a, b

▪ Brachialis Muscle (Figs. 19.45, 19.46, 19.47)

Origin

Surface of the humerus (distal half)

Insertion

- Ulnar tuberosity
- Coronoid process

Action

Flexion in the elbow joint

Innervation

- Musculocutaneous nerve (C5–C6)
- Radial nerve (C7)

Trigger Point Location

TP1   Several centimeters above the inside of the elbow joint

TP2   In the upper half of the muscle belly

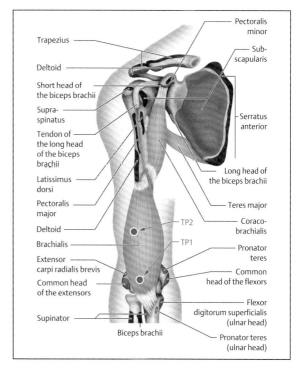

Fig. 19.45

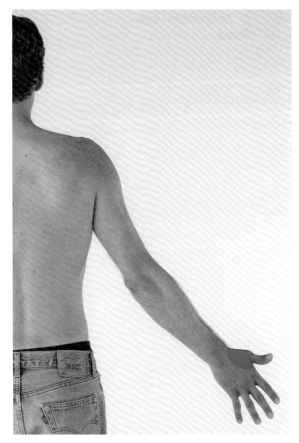

Fig. 19.46

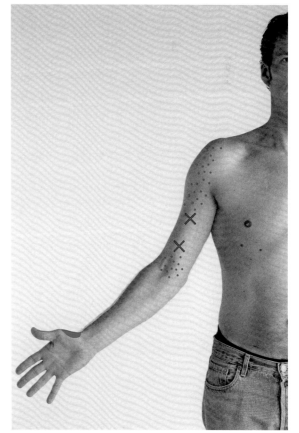

Fig. 19.47

Referred Pain

- Back of the hand in the area of the carpometacarpal joint 1 and base of the thumb

- Inside of the elbow joint
- Ventral upper arm and deltoid area

Associated Internal Organs

None

■ Triceps Brachii Muscle (Figs. 19.48, 19.49)

Origin

- Long head: infraglenoid tubercle of the scapula
- Lateral head: backside of the humerus (proximal half)
- Medial head: backside of the humerus (distal half), inferomedial to the groove for the radial nerve

Insertion

- Olecranon
- Elbow joint capsule

Action

- Extension in the elbow
- Shoulder joint stabilizer

Innervation

Radial nerve (C7–C8)

Trigger Point Location

TP1   In the long head, a few centimeters distal of the place where the teres major crosses over the long triceps head

TP2   In the medial head ca. 4–6 cm above the lateral epicondyle on the lateral edge of the muscle

TP3   In the lateral head on the lateral edge of the muscle around the middle of the upper arm, that is, at the level of the palpation point for the radial nerve on the dorsal upper arm

TP4   In the medial head approximately above the olecranon

TP5   On the medial border of the medial head, a little above the medial epicondyle

Referred Pain

TP1   Dorsal upper arm
Dorsal shoulder region up to the neck
Dorsal forearm up to the back of the hand (with the exception of the elbow)

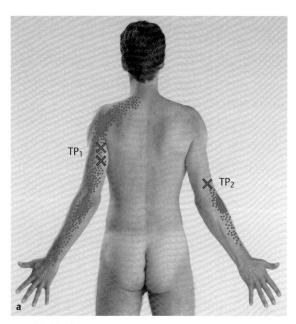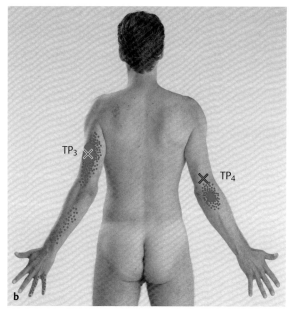

Fig. 19.48a, b

TP2 Lateral epicondyle
      Radial forearm
TP3 Dorsal upper arm
      Dorsal forearm
TP4 Olecranon
TP5 Medial epicondyle
      Ventromedial forearm
      Fingers 4 and 5 palmar

Associated Internal Organs

None

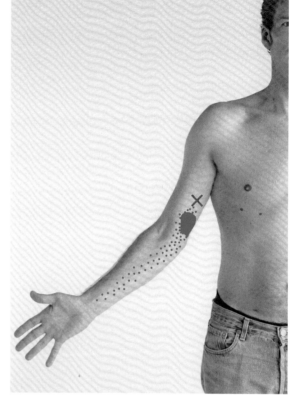

Fig. 19.49

▪ Anconeus Muscle (Fig. 19.50)

Origin

Lateral epicondyle of the humerus (dorsal side)

Insertion

Elbow joint capsule

Action

Tensor of the joint capsule (prevents the joint capsule from getting caught during extension of the elbow)

Innervation

Radial nerve (C6–C8)

Trigger Point Location

Approximately distal of the annular ligament of the radius (see also **Fig. 19.40**)

Referred Pain

Lateral epicondyle

Associated Internal Organs

None

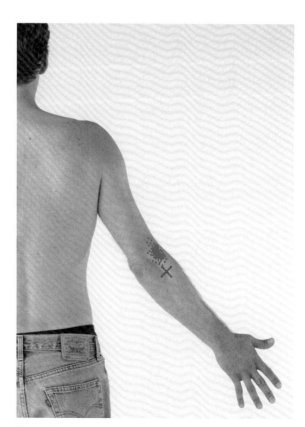

Fig. 19.50

19.3   Muscles of Elbow–Finger Pain

■ Brachioradialis Muscle and Wrist Extensors

Brachioradialis Muscle
(Figs. 19.51, 19.52)

Origin

* Supracondylar crest of the humerus (upper two-thirds)
* Lateral intermuscular septum

Insertion

Styloid process of the radius

Action

* Flexion in the elbow joint
* Brings the forearm into medium position between supination and pronation

Innervation

Radial nerve (C5–C6)

Trigger Point Location

1–2 cm distal of the radius head on the radial side of the forearm approximately in the middle of the muscle belly

Referred Pain

* Back of the hand in the area between the saddle joint of the thumb and the basal joint of the index finger
* Lateral epicondyle
* Radial forearm

Associated Internal Organs

None

Extensor Carpi Radialis Longus Muscle (Fig. 19.53)

Origin

* Lateral supracondylar ridge of the humerus (distal third)
* Lateral intermuscular septum

Insertion

Base of the metacarpal bone II (stretch side)

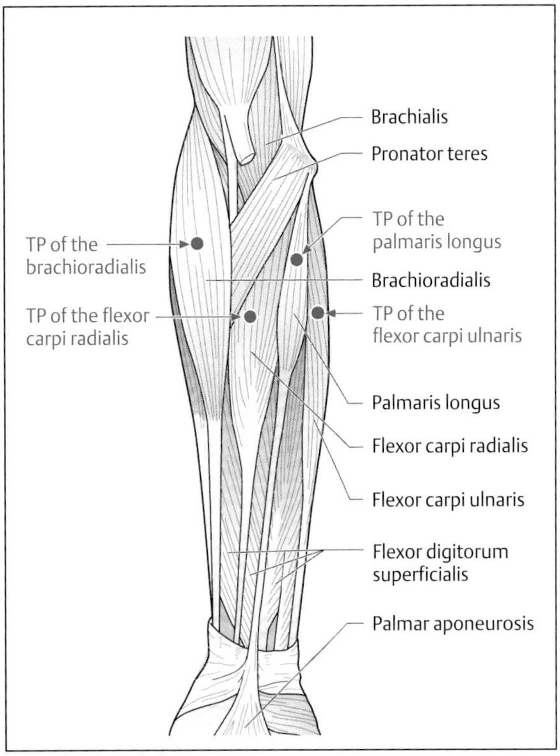

Brachialis

Pronator teres

TP of the palmaris longus

Brachioradialis

TP of the brachioradialis

TP of the flexor carpi ulnaris

TP of the flexor carpi radialis

Palmaris longus

Flexor carpi radialis

Flexor carpi ulnaris

Flexor digitorum superficialis

Palmar aponeurosis

Fig. 19.51

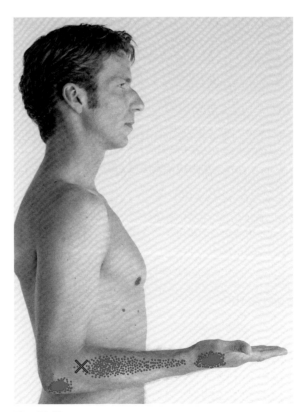

Fig. 19.52

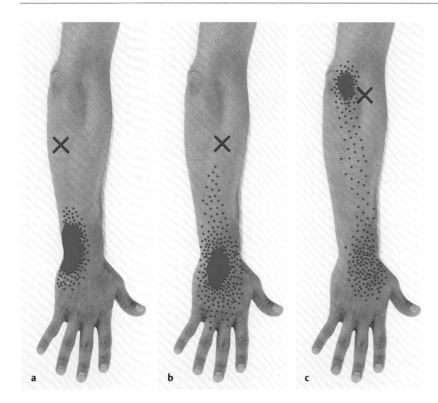

a   b   c

Fig. 19.53a–c

Action

Dorsal extension and radial abduction in the wrist

Innervation

Radial nerve (C6–C7)

Trigger Point Location

1–2 cm distal of the radius head, approximately at the height of the trigger point of the brachioradialis, but further ulnar

Referred Pain

- Lateral epicondyle
- Radial half of the wrist and back of the hand in the area of the metacarpal bones I–III

Associated Internal Organs

None

Extensor Carpi Radialis Brevis Muscle

Origin

Lateral epicondyle of the humerus (front side)

Insertion

Base of the metacarpal bone II (stretch side)

Action

Dorsal extension and radial abduction in the wrist

Innervation

Radial nerve (C7–C8)

Trigger Point Location

Approximately 5–6 cm distal from the radius head (roughly in the middle of the muscle belly) (see **Fig. 19. 53**)

Referred Pain

Central area of the wrist and back of the hand

Associated Internal Organs

None

Extensor Carpi Ulnaris Muscle

Origin

Lateral epicondyle of the humerus (front side)

Insertion

Base of the metacarpal bone V

Action

Dorsal extension and ulnar abduction in the wrist

Innervation

Radial nerve (C7–C8)

Trigger Point Location

Approximately 7–8 cm distal from the lateral epicondyle (see **Figs. 19.53** and **19.55**)

Referred Pain

Ulnar half of the wrist

Associated Internal Organs

None

▪ Extensor Digitorum and Indicis Muscles

Extensor Digitorum Muscle (Figs. 19.54, 19.55)

Origin

Lateral epicondyle of the humerus (front side)

Insertion

Middle and end phalanges of fingers 2–5 (indirectly by radiating the four muscle tendons into the dorsal aponeurosis)

Action

Extension of the finger joints

Innervation

Radial nerve (C7–C8)

Trigger Point Location

- Trigger point for the middle finger: 3–4 cm distal and somewhat dorsal of the radius head
- Trigger points for the ring and little finger lie a little distal from there, deep in the muscle belly

Referred Pain

- Lateral epicondyle (sometimes included when ring or little finger are affected)
- Dorsal forearm
- Wrist
- Back of the hand
- Fingers, except for the end phalanx

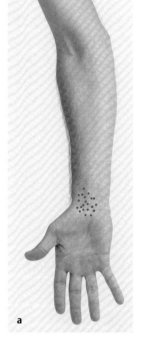
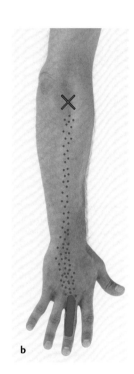

a   b

Fig. 19.54a, b

The referred pain is felt in different fingers, depending on the position of the trigger point.

Associated Internal Organs

None

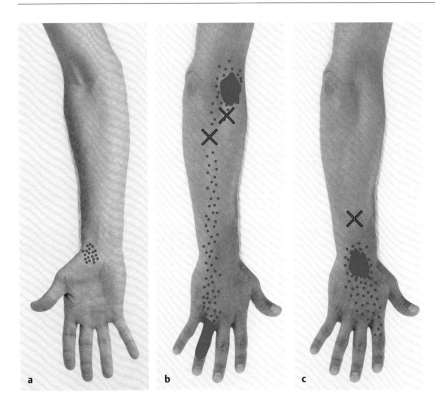

Fig. 19.55a–c

Extensor Indicis Muscle (Fig. 19.56)

Origin

• Backside of the ulna (distal section)
• Interosseous membrane

Insertion

Radiates into the dorsal aponeurosis of the index finger

Action

Extension of the index finger

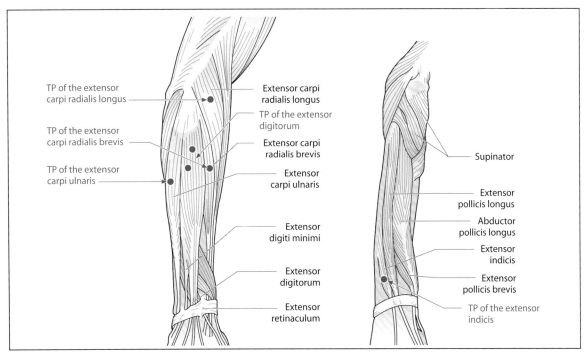

Fig. 19.56

Innervation

Radial nerve (C7–C8)

Trigger Point Location

In the distal half of the muscle in the middle of the forearm between the radius and ulna (see **Fig. 19.55**)

Referred Pain

Radial side of the wrist and back of hand

Associated Internal Organs

None

■ Supinator Muscle (Figs. 19.57, 19.58, 19.59)

Origin

- Supinator crest of the ulna
- Lateral epicondyle of the humerus
- Radial collateral ligament
- Annular ligament of the radius

Insertion

Neck and shaft of the radius (between the tuberosity of the radius and the insertion of the pronator teres)

Action

Supination of the forearm

Innervation

Radial nerve

Trigger Point Location

Slightly lateral and distal of the biceps tendon in the superficial part of the muscle on the ventral side of the radius

Referred Pain

- Lateral epicondyle and in the lateral area of the elbow
- Dorsal back of the hand between the metacarpal bones I and II
- Dorsal proximal phalanx of the thumb

Associated Internal Organs

None

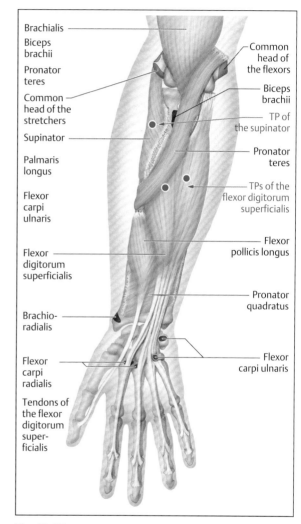

Fig. 19.57

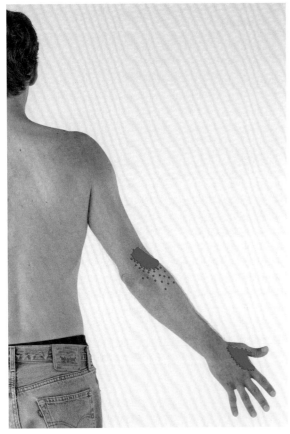

Fig. 19.58

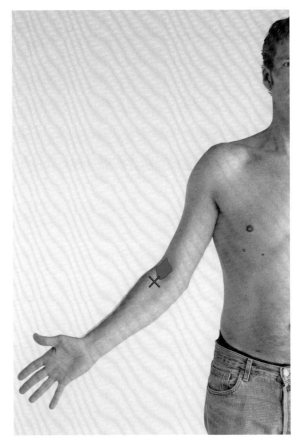

Fig. 19.59

▪ Palmaris Longus Muscle (Fig. 19.60)

Origin

Medial epicondyle of the humerus

Insertion

• Flexor retinaculum
• Palmar aponeurosis

Action

Stretching the palmar aponeurosis

Innervation

Median nerve (C7–C8)

Trigger Point Location

At the transition from the proximal to the medial third of the ventral forearm

Referred Pain

• Palm of the hand
• Distal half of the anterior forearm

Associated Internal Organs

None

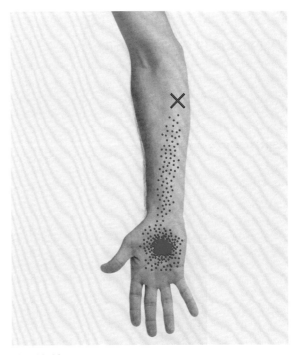

Fig. 19.60

■ Flexor Carpi Radialis and Ulnaris, Flexor Digitorum Superficialis and Profundus, Flexor Pollicis Longus, and Pronator Teres Muscles

Flexor Carpi Radialis Muscle (Fig. 19.61a1)

Origin

Medial epicondyle of the humerus

Insertion

• Base of the metacarpal bones II and III
• Scaphoid bone

Action

• Palmar flexion
• Radial abduction

Innervation

Median nerve (C6–C7)

Trigger Point Location

In the center of the muscle belly (in the center of the ventral forearm in the proximal half)

Referred Pain

• Ventral wrist area between the thenar and the hypothenar eminence
• Proximal half of the palm
• Narrow band in the distal half of the forearm

Associated Internal Organs

None

Flexor Carpi Ulnaris Muscle (Fig. 19.61a2)

Origin

• Medial epicondyle of the humerus
• Olecranon
• Posterior border of the ulna
• Antebrachial fascia

Insertion

• Piriform bone
• Hook of hamate bone
• Via the pisohamate and pisometacarpal ligaments at the base of the metacarpal bone V

Action

• Palmar flexion
• Ulnar abduction

Innervation

Ulnar nerve (C6–C7)

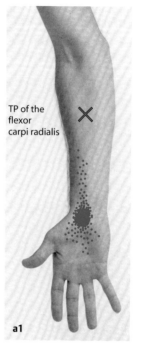

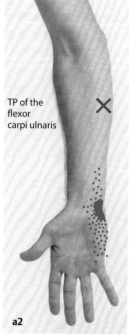

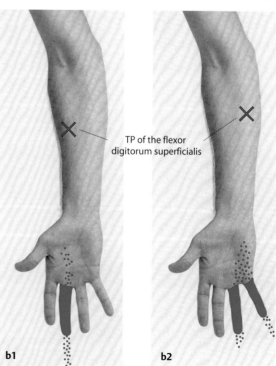

Fig. 19.61a, b

Trigger Point Location

In the center of the muscle belly at the ulnar rim of the ventral forearm in the proximal half (see **Figs. 19.51** and **19.61**)

Referred Pain

- Ventral wrist area in the area of the ulnar edge of the hypothenar eminence
- Proximal half of the palm (hypothenar area)
- Narrow band in the distal half of the forearm (hypothenar area)

Associated Internal Organs

None

Flexor Digitorum Superficialis Muscle
(Fig. 19.61b1, b2)

Origin

- Medial epicondyle of the humerus (up to the medial collateral ligaments of the elbow)
- Coronoid process of the ulna (medial rim)
- Oblique cord
- Front side of the radius along the oblique line

Insertion

Laterally at the medial phalanges of fingers 2–5

Action

- Flexion of the intermediate and proximal joints of fingers 2–5
- Flexion in the wrist

Innervation

Median nerve (C7–C8) (see **Fig. 19.57**)

Flexor Digitorum Profundus Muscle
(Fig. 19.62)

Origin

- Olecranon (medial)
- Anterior and medial side of the ulna
- Interosseous membrane

Insertion

Distal phalanx of fingers 2–5

Action

- Flexion of all finger joints
- Flexion of the wrist

Innervation

- Median nerve (C6–C7)
- Ulnar nerve (C7–C8)

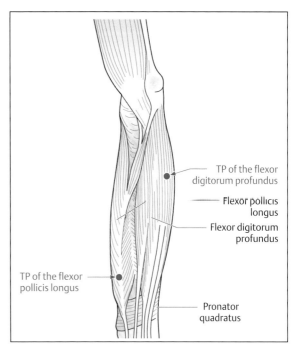

Fig. 19.62

Trigger Point Location for Both Muscles

Ventral forearm in the proximal half on one line with the trigger points of the flexor carpi radialis and ulnaris (see **Fig. 19.61a1, a2**)

Referred Pain for Both Muscles

Plantar side of fingers 3–5 (they can also hurt individually).

Associated Internal Organs

None

Flexor Pollicis Longus Muscle (Fig. 19.62)

Origin

- Anterior fascia of the radius (distal to the oblique line)
- Interosseous membrane

Insertion

Base of the distal phalanx of the thumb

Action

Flexion of the thumb's distal phalanx

Innervation

Median nerve (C7–C8)

Trigger Point Location

Slightly proximal of the wrist and radial of the median line of the forearm

Referred Pain

Ventral side of the thumb

Associated Internal Organs

None

Pronator Teres Muscle (Fig. 19.63)

Origin

• Medial epicondyle of the humerus
• Medial intermuscular septum
• Coronoid process of the ulna

Insertion

Pronator tuberosity

Action

• Pronation of the forearm
• Flexion in the elbow joint

Innervation

Median nerve (C6–C7)

Trigger Point Location

Near the inside of the elbow, ulnar to the bicipital apo-neurosis of the biceps brachii (see **Fig. 19.40**)

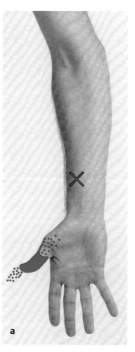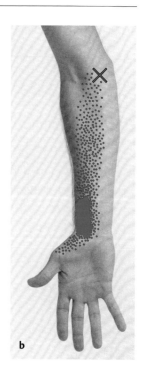

Fig. 19.63a, b

Referred Pain

• Ventral and radial area of the wrist
• Radial, ventral half of the forearm

Associated Internal Organs

None

■ Adductor and Opponens Pollicis Muscles

Adductor Pollicis Muscle
(Figs. 19.64, 19.65)

Origin

• Base of the metacarpal bones II–III
• Trapezoid bone
• Capitate bone
• Body of the metacarpal bone III

Insertion

• Ulnar sesamoid bone
• Proximal phalanx of the thumb (ulnar side)
• Tendon of the extensor pollicis longus

Action

Adduction of the thumb

Innervation

Ulnar nerve (T1)

Trigger Point Location

Near the skin fold between the thumb and index finger in the muscle belly. Easily palpated with a pinching grip.

Referred Pain

• Radial side of the base joint of the thumb up to the thumb's saddle joint
• Thenar eminence
• Dorsal back of the hand in the area of the thumb

Associated Internal Organs

None

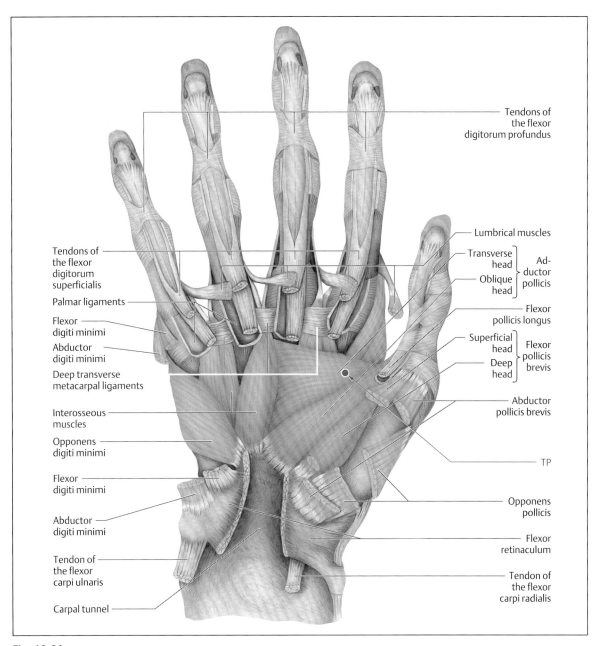

Tendons of
the flexor
digitorum profundus

Lumbrical muscles

Transverse
head ⎫
        ⎬ Ad-
Oblique ⎪ ductor
head ⎭ pollicis

Flexor
pollicis longus

Superficial ⎫
head ⎬ Flexor
        ⎪ pollicis
Deep ⎭ brevis
head

Abductor
pollicis brevis

TP

Opponens
pollicis

Flexor
retinaculum

Tendon of
the flexor
carpi radialis

Tendons of
the flexor
digitorum
superficialis

Palmar ligaments

Flexor
digiti minimi

Abductor
digiti minimi

Deep transverse
metacarpal ligaments

Interosseous
muscles

Opponens
digiti minimi

Flexor
digiti minimi

Abductor
digiti minimi

Tendon of
the flexor
carpi ulnaris

Carpal tunnel

Fig. 19.64

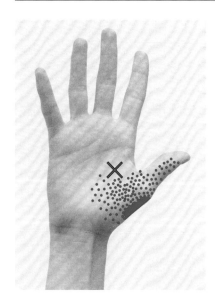
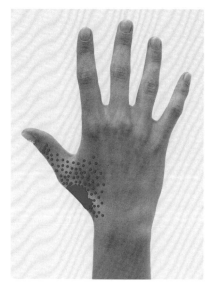

Fig. 19.65

Opponens Pollicis Muscle (Fig. 19.66)

Origin

• Flexor retinaculum
• Tubercle of trapezium bone

Insertion

Metacarpal bone I (radial)

Action

Opposition of the thumb

Innervation

• Median nerve (C8–T1)
• Ulnar nerve (T1)

Trigger Point Location

In the muscle belly near the wrist

Referred Pain

• Palmar side of the thumb
• Radial and plantar half of the wrist

Associated Internal Organs

None

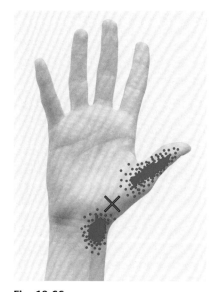

Fig. 19.66

▪ Abductor Digiti Minimi Muscle (Figs. 19.67, 19.68)

Origin

Pisiform bone

Insertion

Ulnar base of the proximal phalanx and dorsal apo-neurosis of finger 5

Action

- Flexion and abduction in the proximal joint of the little finger
- Extension in the intermediate and distal joints of the little finger

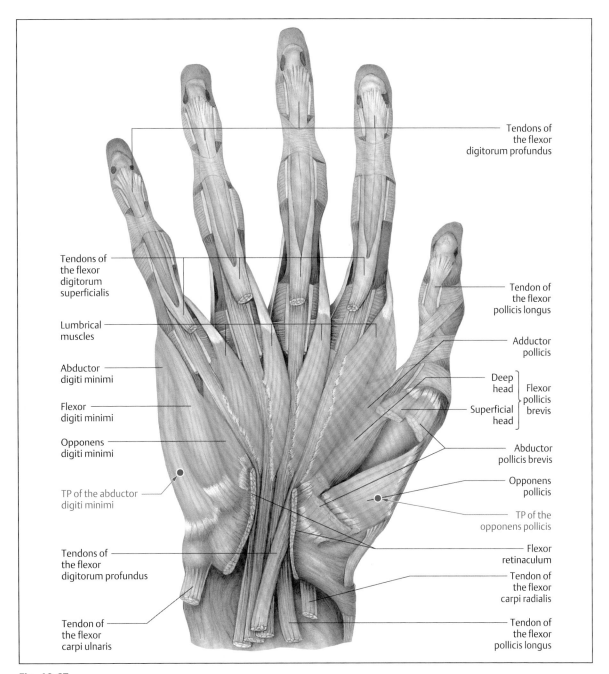

Tendons of the flexor digitorum profundus

Tendons of the flexor digitorum superficialis

Lumbrical muscles

Abductor digiti minimi

Flexor digiti minimi

Opponens digiti minimi

TP of the abductor digiti minimi

Tendons of the flexor digitorum profundus

Tendon of the flexor carpi ulnaris

Tendon of the flexor pollicis longus

Adductor pollicis

Deep head ⎤
⎥ Flexor
⎥ pollicis
Superficial ⎥ brevis
head ⎦

Abductor pollicis brevis

Opponens pollicis

TP of the opponens pollicis

Flexor retinaculum

Tendon of the flexor carpi radialis

Tendon of the flexor pollicis longus

Fig. 19.67

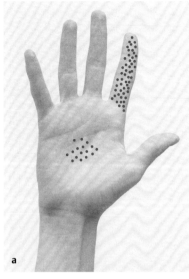
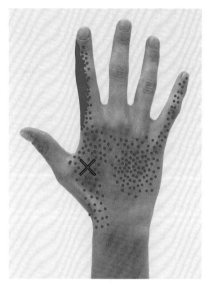
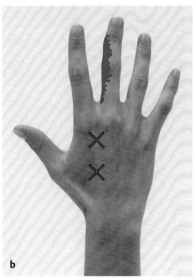
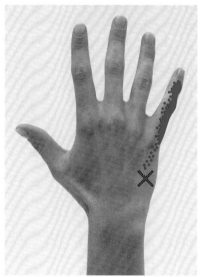

Fig. 19.68a, b

Innervation

Ulnar nerve (C8–T1)

Trigger Point Location

In the muscle belly near the base of the metacarpal bone V

Referred Pain

Ulnar side of the little finger

Associated Internal Organs

None

■ Interosseous Muscles (Fig. 19.69)

Dorsal Interosseous Muscles

Origin

Inside of all metacarpal bones

Insertion

• Base of the corresponding proximal phalanges
• Dorsal aponeurosis of fingers 2–4

Action

• Abduction of fingers 2–4
• Flexion of the proximal joints of the fingers with extension of the intermediate and distal joints

Innervation

Ulnar nerve (T1)

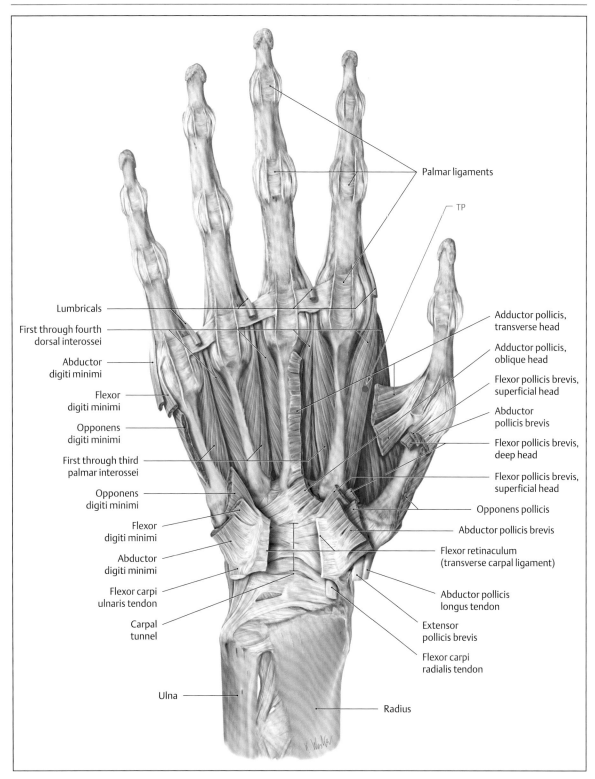

Palmar ligaments

TP

Lumbricals

First through fourth
dorsal interossei

Abductor
digiti minimi

Flexor
digiti minimi

Opponens
digiti minimi

First through third
palmar interossei

Opponens
digiti minimi

Flexor
digiti minimi

Abductor
digiti minimi

Flexor carpi
ulnaris tendon

Carpal
tunnel

Ulna

Adductor pollicis,
transverse head

Adductor pollicis,
oblique head

Flexor pollicis brevis,
superficial head

Abductor
pollicis brevis

Flexor pollicis brevis,
deep head

Flexor pollicis brevis,
superficial head

Opponens pollicis

Abductor pollicis brevis

Flexor retinaculum
(transverse carpal ligament)

Abductor pollicis
longus tendon

Extensor
pollicis brevis

Flexor carpi
radialis tendon

Radius

Fig. 19.69   **From:** *Thieme Atlas of Anatomy, Vol. I: General Anatomy and Musculoskeletal System.* Thieme Publishers, Stuttgart 2006.

Palmar Interosseous Muscles

Origin

Metacarpal bones II, IV, and V

Insertion

- Base of the corresponding proximal phalanges
- Radiating into the tendons of the dorsal aponeurosis of fingers 2, 4, and 5
- Ulnar sesamoid bone of the thumb

Action

- Adduction of the fingers 2, 4, and 5
- Flexion of the proximal joints of the fingers with extension of the intermediate and distal joints

Innervation

Ulnar nerve (T1)

Trigger Point Location

Between the metacarpal bones (see **Fig. 19.68**)

Referred Pain

- Index finger (with a maximum on the radial side) and back of the hand (trigger point of the dorsal interosseous muscles of the index finger, a very common trigger point)
- Radial side of the fingers

Associated Internal Organs

None

19.4   Muscles of Upper Torso Pain

■ Pectoralis Major Muscle (Fig. 19.70)

Origin

- Clavicular part:
  - clavicle (sternal half)
- Sternocostal part:
  - lateral at the manubrium and body of the sternum
  - rib cartilage 1–6
  - aponeurosis of the abdominal external oblique muscle

Insertion

- Crest of the lesser tubercle of the humerus
- Deltoid tuberosity (ventral)

Action

- Clavicular part: flexion, adduction in the shoulder joint
- Sternocostal part: adduction and internal rotation in the shoulder joint, inhalatory muscle

Innervation

Medial and lateral pectoral nerves (C6–C8)

Trigger Point Location

Trigger points are distributed throughout the entire muscle. The points that are located more laterally and closer to the armpit are easily found by pinching palpation. The more sternally located points are detected by shallow palpation.

Trigger point of "arrhythmia": In the center between two vertical lines, of which one runs through the nipple and the other through the lateral border of the sternum, look for the trigger point in the intercostal space between the fifth and sixth rib on the right side.

Referred Pain

Trigger points of the clavicular part:
- Ventral deltoid area
- Clavicular part itself

Trigger points of the sternocostal part, lateral:
- Ventral chest area
- On the inside of the upper arm
- Medial epicondyle
- Ventral forearm
- Ulnar edge of hand
- Palmar hand surface of fingers 3–5

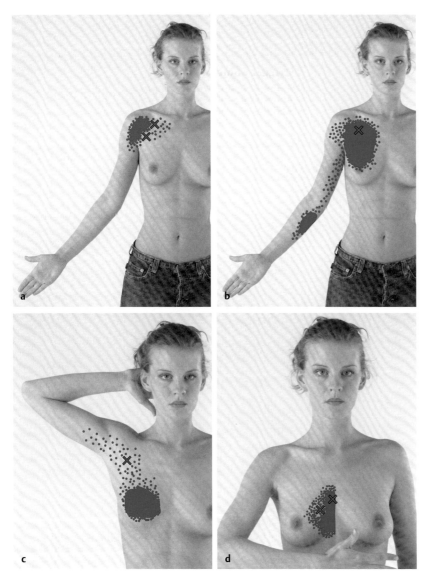

Fig. 19.70a–d

Trigger points of the sternocostal part, medial:
- Sternum (without crossing over the center line) and bordering chest area

Trigger points of the sternocostal part, caudal:
- Ventral chest area with hypersensitivity in the nipple and possibly in the entire chest (especially in women)

Trigger points of "arrhythmia":
- This trigger point occurs in cardial arrhythmia without causing pain.

Associated Internal Organs

Heart

■ Pectoralis Minor Muscle (Fig. 19.71)

Origin

Third to fifth rib

Insertion

Coronoid process of the scapula (cranial-medial)

Action

• Pulls the scapula forward and downward
• Inhalatory muscle when shoulder blade is fixed

Innervation

Medial and lateral pectoral nerves (C6–C8)

Trigger Point Location

TP1 Near the origin of the muscle at the fourth rib
TP2 At the transition from the muscle belly to the tendon slightly caudal from the coronoid process of the scapula

Referred Pain

• Ventral deltoid area
• Chest area
• Ulnar side of the upper arm, elbow, forearm
• Palmar hand surface of fingers 3–5

The referred pain pattern closely resembles that of the pectoralis major.

Associated Internal Organs

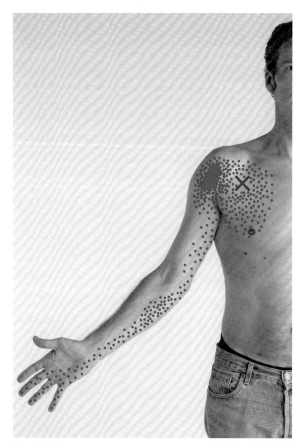

Fig. 19.71

Heart

■ Subclavius Muscle (Figs. 19.72, 19.73)

Origin

First rib (cartilage-bone border)

Insertion

Clavicle in the middle third on the underside

Action

Pulls the clavicle downward

Innervation

Subclavian nerve (C5–C6)

Trigger Point Location

Near the insertion of the muscle

Referred Pain

• Ventral area of the shoulder and upper arm
• Radial side of the forearm
• Palmar and dorsal hand surface in the area of fingers 1–3

Associated Internal Organs

The subclavius is frequently innervated by a branch of the phrenic nerve. This leads to connections with the:
• Liver
• Gallbladder

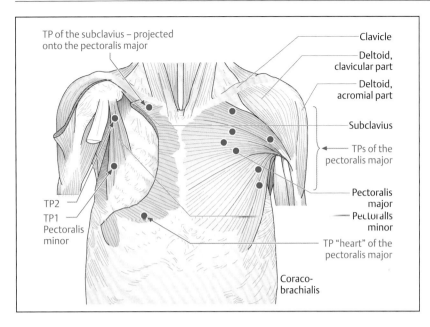

TP of the subclavius – projected onto the pectoralis major

Clavicle

Deltoid, clavicular part

Deltoid, acromial part

Subclavius

TPs of the pectoralis major

Pectoralis major

Pectoralis minor

TP2

TP1 Pectoralis minor

TP "heart" of the pectoralis major

Coraco-brachialis

Fig. 19.72

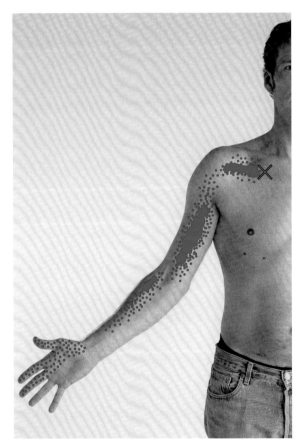

Fig. 19.73

▪ Sternalis Muscle (Fig. 19.74)

Only found in one out of 20 people.

Origin

Unilaterally or bilaterally in the pectoral fascia or the fascia of the SCM with possible origins in the cranial sternum area

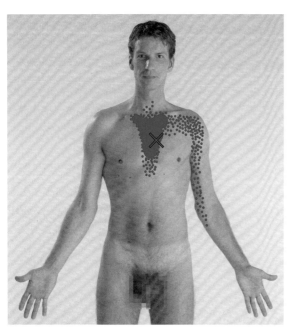

Fig. 19.74

Insertion

Great variability with possible insertions between the third to seventh rib cartilage, pectoral fascia, or the fascia of the rectus abdominis

Action

Unknown, possibly fascia stretcher

Innervation

Medial pectoral nerve (C6–C8) or intercostal nerves

Trigger Point Location

Trigger points can be found in the entire muscle belly, mostly in the central area of the sternum.

Referred Pain

* Entire sternum, possibly also substernal
* Upper chest area
* Ventral upper arm and elbow

The referred pain pattern resembles the pain of a heart attack or angina pectoris.

Associated Internal Organs

Heart

▪ Serratus Posterior Superior Muscle (Figs. 19.75, 19.76)

Origin

Spinous process and supraspinous ligaments of C7–T2

Insertion

Outside of ribs 2–5 (posterior)

Action

Inhalatory muscle in deep inhalation

Innervation

Ventral branches of the spinal nerves T2–T5

Trigger Point Location

In neutral position, the trigger point projects itself at the height of the supraspinatous scapular fossa near the scapular spine onto the dorsal wall of the torso.

Referred Pain

* Underneath the scapula in its upper half
* Dorsal deltoid area
* Dorsal upper arm
* Ulnar side of the forearm
* Elbow, dorsal
* Ventral and dorsal surface of the hand in the area of the hypothenar eminence and finger 5
* Pectoral area

Associated Internal Organs

* Heart
* Lung

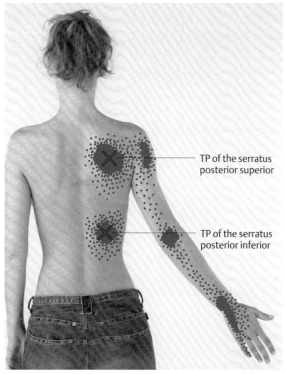

TP of the serratus posterior superior

TP of the serratus posterior inferior

Fig. 19.75

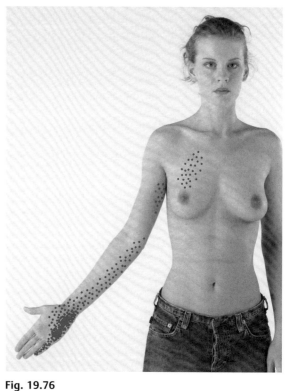

Fig. 19.76

▪ Serratus Posterior Inferior Muscle (Fig. 19.77)

Origin

Spinous process and supraspinous ligaments of T11–L2

Insertion

Outside of ribs 9–12 (posterior)

Action

Exhalatory muscle in deep exhalation

Innervation

Ventral branches of the spinal nerves T9–T12

Trigger Point Location

In the muscle belly near the insertion to the ribs (see **Fig. 19.75**)

Referred Pain

In the area of the muscle around the lower ribs

Associated Internal Organs

- Kidneys
- Duodenum
- Pancreas
- Jejunum, ilium
- Colon
- Uterus

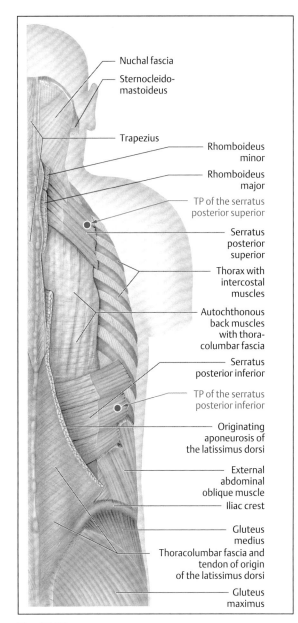

Nuchal fascia

Sternocleido-
mastoideus

Trapezius

Rhomboideus
minor

Rhomboideus
major

TP of the serratus
posterior superior

Serratus
posterior
superior

Thorax with
intercostal
muscles

Autochthonous
back muscles
with thora-
columbar fascia

Serratus
posterior inferior

TP of the serratus
posterior inferior

Originating
aponeurosis of
the latissimus dorsi

External
abdominal
oblique muscle

Iliac crest

Gluteus
medius

Thoracolumbar fascia and
tendon of origin
of the latissimus dorsi

Gluteus
maximus

Fig. 19.77

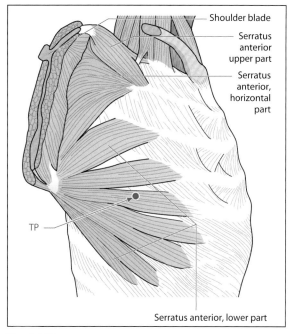

Shoulder blade

Serratus
anterior
upper part

Serratus
anterior,
horizontal
part

TP

Serratus anterior, lower part

Fig. 19.78

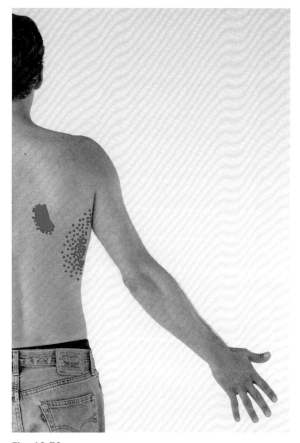

Fig. 19.79

■ Serratus Anterior Muscle

(Figs. 19.78, 19.79, 19.80, 19.81)

Origin

Ribs 1–9 and intercostal spaces in the area of the
medioclavicular line

Insertion

Medial border of the scapula

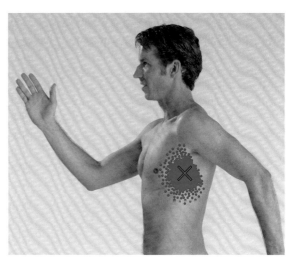

Fig. 19.81

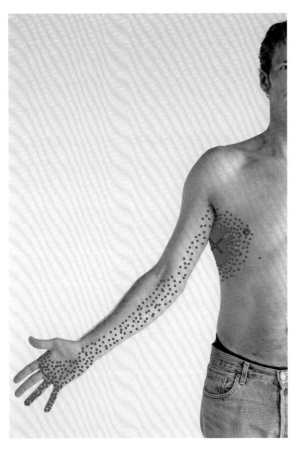

Fig. 19.80

Action

- Pulls the scapula to ventrolateral
- Accessory muscle of inhalation

Innervation

- Long thoracic nerve (C5–C7)
- Intercostal nerves

Trigger Point Location

In the muscle shaft that originates at the fifth or sixth rib, near the middle axillary line

Referred Pain

- Anterolateral in the central chest area
- Medial from the lower scapula angle
- Medial upper and forearm
- Hand surface with fingers 4 and 5

Deepened breathing, such as during sports, can cause pain like stitches in the side

Associated Internal Organs

Heart

■ Erector Spinae Muscles (Figs. 19.82, 19.83, 19.84)

Iliocostal Muscle

Origin

- Sacral bone
- Iliac crest
- Spinous processes of the lumbar spinal column (LSC)
- Thoracolumbar fascia
- Costal angle

Insertion

Cranial and caudal at the transverse processes of the middle CSC or rib angles for the lumbar and thoracic area

Action

- Lateral flexion of the spinal column
- Extension of the spinal column

Innervation

Dorsal branches of the segmental spinal nerves

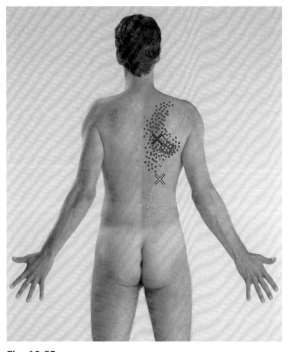

Fig. 19.82

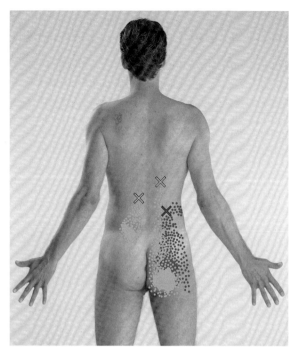

Fig. 19.83

Longissimus Muscle

Origin

- Transverse processes
- Sacral bone
- Iliac crest
- Spinous and mammillary processes of the LSC

Insertion

- Transverse processes that are located cranial from the origin
- Mastoid process
- Costal and accessory process of ribs 2–12

Action

Extension of the spinal column

Innervation

Dorsal branches of the segmental spinal nerves

Spinalis Muscle

Origin

Spinous processes of the spinal column

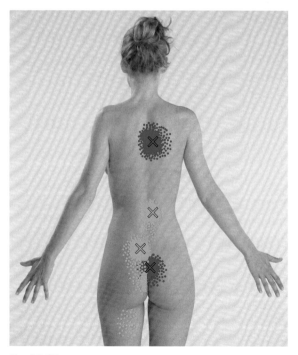

Fig. 19.84

Insertion

Spinous processes of the six vertebrae that lie cranial to the origin

Action

Lateral flexion of the spinal column

Innervation

Dorsal branches of the segmental spinal nerves

Trigger Point Location

Trigger points can be distributed all throughout the erector spinae muscles. It is helpful in finding the trigger points that the spinous processes may be hypersensitive at the height where the erector spinae trigger points are active.

Referred Pain

- Trigger points in the iliocostalis, central thorax area: To cranial into the shoulder area and into the lateral chest wall.
- Trigger points in the iliocostalis, lower thorax area: To cranial above the scapula, forward into the abdomen and into the upper LSC.

- Trigger points in the iliocostalis, lumbar section: To caudal in the central buttocks area.
- Trigger points in the longissimus: Into the gluteal area and the iliosacral joint (ISJ) region.
- Trigger points in the spinalis: The pain is concentrated around the trigger point.

Associated Internal Organs

- Jejunum, ilium
- Colon
- Kidneys
- Urinary bladder
- Uterus
- Ovaries
- Prostate

▪ Rectus Abdominis, Abdominal Internal and External Oblique, Transversus Abdominis, and Pyramidalis Muscles (Figs. 19.85, 19.86, 19.87, 19.88)

Rectus Abdominis Muscle

Origin

- Pubic crest
- Pubic symphysis

Insertion

- Fifth to seventh rib cartilage
- Rib arch, medial area
- Xyphoid process, backside

Action

- Torso flexion
- Abdominal press
- Forced exhalation

Innervation

Ventral branches of the spinal nerves T7–T12

Abdominal Internal Oblique Muscle

Origin

- Thoracolumbar fascia
- Frontal two-thirds of the iliac crest
- Lateral two-thirds of the inguinal ligament

Insertion

- Rib arch
- Anterior and posterior lamina of the rectus sheath
- Tendinous to the pubic crest and pectineal line

Action

- Sidebend of the torso
- Rotation of the torso to the ipsilateral side (together with the contralateral muscle)

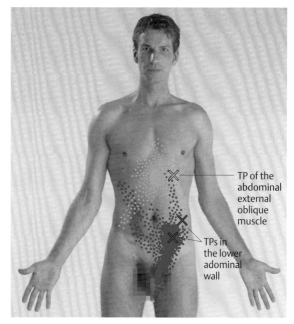

TP of the abdominal external oblique muscle

TPs in the lower adominal wall

Fig. 19.85

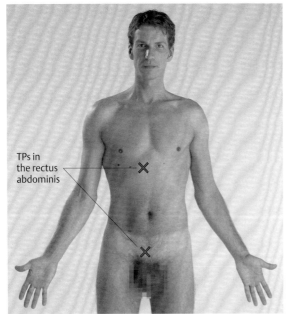

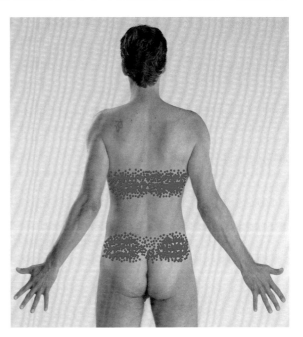

Fig. 19.86

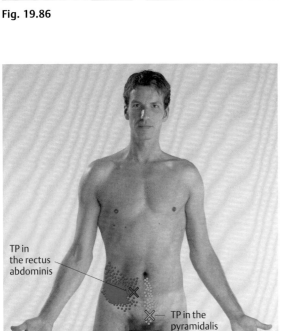

Fig. 19.87

- Abdominal press
- Forced exhalation
- Reinforcement of the inguinal canal

Innervation

Ventral branches of the spinal nerves T7–T12

Abdominal External Oblique Muscle

Origin

Ventral outside of ribs 5–12

Insertion

- Iliac crest
- Inguinal ligament
- Pubic tubercle
- Pubic crest
- Linea alba

Action

- Sidebend of the torso
- Rotation of the torso to the contralateral side (together with contralateral muscle)
- Abdominal press
- Forced exhalation

Innervation

Ventral branches of the spinal nerves T7–T12

Transversus Abdominis Muscle

Origin

- Inside of the lower ribs
- Thoracolumbar fascia
- Frontal two-thirds of the iliac crest
- Outer half of the inguinal ligament

Insertion

- Anterior and posterior lamina of the rectus sheath
- Pubic crest
- Pecten pubis

Action

- Abdominal press
- Forced exhalation
- Reinforcement of the inguinal canal

Innervation

Ventral branches of the spinal nerves T7–T12

Pyramidalis Muscle

Origin

Pubic crest, ventral from the insertion of the rectus abdominis

Insertion

Linea alba, distal

Action

Reinforcement of the rectus sheath

Innervation

Subcostal nerve (T12)

Abdominal Muscles

Trigger Point Location

We find trigger points distributed throughout the entire abdominal musculature. **Figs. 19.85–19.88** demonstrate a selection of common trigger point localizations.

Referred Pain

In general, we can state that a majority of trigger points in the abdominal muscles have in common that they generate mostly localized pain around the trigger point. In addition, trigger points in the abdominal muscles cause a number of visceral symptoms, such as nausea, vomiting, or dysmenorrhea. A further special characteristic of trigger points in the abdominal musclesis that the referred pain crosses over the center line. Nevertheless, we can define a few typical pain patterns for the abdominal muscles:

***Trigger points for the externus abdominis,
rib section:***
- "Heart pain"
- Symptoms resembling a hiatal hernia

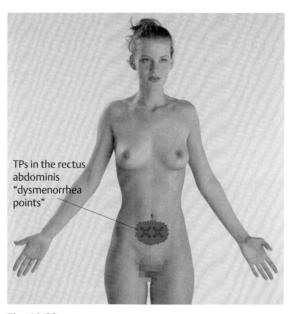

TPs in the rectus abdominis "dysmenorrhea points"

Fig. 19.88

- Epigastric pain that extends to other abdominal regions

Trigger points of the lower abdominal wall (all muscles of the abdominal wall):
- Pain in the groin and testicles or labia
- Other sections of the abdomen

Trigger points along the upper rim of the pubic bone and the lateral half of the inguinal ligament (internus and rectus abdominis muscles):
- Pain in the area of the urinary bladder to the point of urinary bladder spasms
- Inguinal pain
- Retention of urine

Trigger points in the transversus abdominis, above the insertion of the ribs:
- Upper abdomen between the arches of the ribs

Trigger points in the rectus abdominis, above the navel:
- Painful band across the back at the height of the thoracolumbar junction (TLJ)

Trigger points in the rectus abdominis, at the height of the navel on the lateral edge of the muscle:
- Abdominal spasms and colic-like pain
- Pain in the ventral abdominal wall without strict pattern

Trigger points in the rectus abdominis, below the navel:
- Dysmenorrhea
- Painful band across the back at the height of the sacrum

Trigger point in the pyramidalis:
- Between the symphysis and the navel, near the center line

Associated Internal Organs

- Liver
- Gall bladder
- Stomach
- Pancreas
- Spleen
- Duodenum
- Jejunum, ilium

- Colon
- Kidneys
- Uterus
- Ovaries

The acute abdomen impresses by firmly tensing the abdominal wall. We can explain this as a segmental viscerosomatic reflex: the abdominal muscles react with a calming hypertonus to the peritoneal irritation of the segmentally associated organ.

After organic disorders are cured, trigger points regularly persist in the abdominal muscles.

19.5   Muscles of Lower Torso Pain

■ Quadratus Lumborum Muscle (Figs. 19.89, 19.90, 19.91)

Origin

Lower rim of the 12th rib

Insertion

- Costal processes of L1–L4
- Iliolumbar ligament
- Posterior third of the iliac crest

Action

- Lateral flexion of the torso
- Fixation of the 12th rib during respiration

Innervation

Ventral branches of the spinal nerves T12–L3

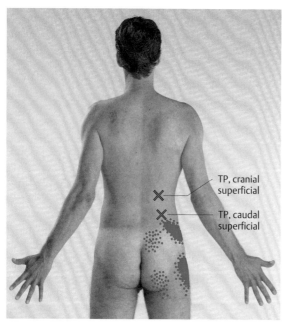

TP, cranial superficial
TP, caudal superficial

Fig. 19.89

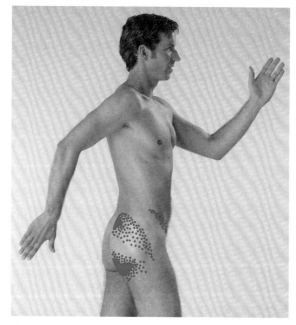

Fig. 19.90

Trigger Point Location

For easier palpation, lie the patient on their contralateral side with a rolled-up towel in the waist, resulting in a sidebend of the spinal column away from the muscle that is to be palpated. The arm that lies on top is placed in maximal abduction and the upper leg is stretched while the leg below is slightly flexed. The desired sidebend is thereby reinforced.

Palpate the following areas of the muscle for trigger points:

• In the angle above the iliac crest and lateral to the erector spinae
• Along the iliac crest
• In the angle between the 12th rib and the erector spinae

The superficial trigger points are found in the lateral areas of the muscle, either below the 12th rib or above the iliac crest.

The deep trigger points are found either above the iliac crest between the costal processes of the fourth and fifth lumbar vertebrae or at the height of the costal processes of the third lumbar vertebra in the medial regions of the muscle.

Referred Pain

• Cranial superficial trigger point: along the iliac crest, sometimes into the groin and the lower lateral abdominal region
• Caudal superficial trigger point: around the trochanter, partly pulling into the lateral thigh
• Cranial deep trigger point: into the area of the ISJ
• Caudal deep trigger point: caudal buttocks

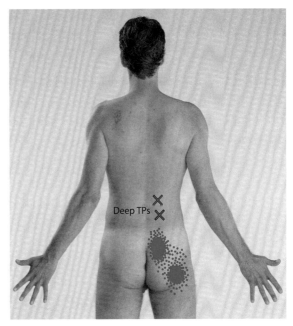

Fig. 19.91

Associated Internal Organs

• Jejunum, ilium
• Colon
• Kidneys
• Urinary bladder
• Uterus, adnexa, prostate

▩ Iliopsoas Muscle (Figs. 19.92, 19.93, 19.94)

Iliacus Muscle

Origin

Iliac fossa

Insertion

Lesser trochanter of the femur

Action

• Flexion in the hip joint
• Outward and internal rotation in the hip joint

Innervation

Femoral nerve (L2–L3)

Psoas Major Muscle

Origin

• Transverse processes of L1–L5
• T12–L5 and the discs below T12

Insertion

Lesser trochanter of the femur

Action

• Flexion in the hip joint
• Outward and internal rotation in the hip joint
• Abduction in the hip joint
• Extension and lateral flexion of the LSC

Innervation

Ventral branches of the spinal nerves L1–L2

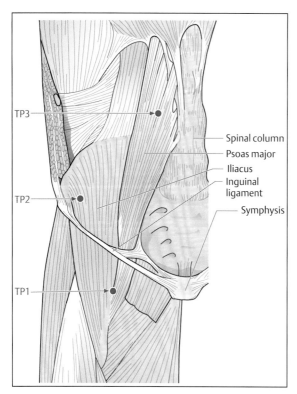

Fig. 19.92

Psoas Minor Muscle

Origin

T12–L1 including disk

Insertion

Iliac fascia

Action

Bending the torso (slight)

Innervation

Ventral branch of the spinal nerve L1

Trigger Point Location

TP1   Lateral border of the femoral triangle

TP2   In the iliac fossa at the height of the anterior superior iliac spine (ASIS)

TP3   Lateral of the rectus abdominis and below the navel. First palpate carefully to posterior and then to medial, to compress the psoas major against the spinal column

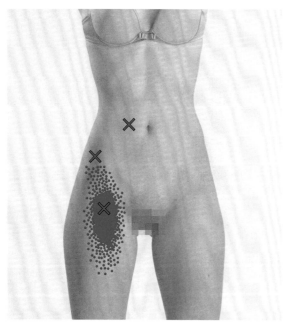

Fig. 19.93

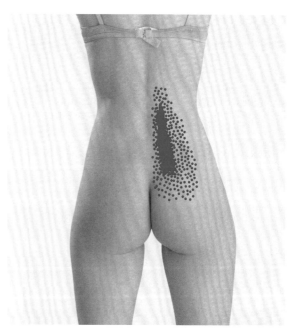

Fig. 19.94

Referred Pain

- Primarily in the LSC ipsilateral along the spinal column up to the ISJ and to the upper to middle buttocks area
- Groin and anteromedial thigh

Associated Internal Organs

- Colon
- Kidneys
- Urinary bladder
- Uterus, adnexa, prostate

■ Muscles of the Pelvic Floor (Figs. 19.95, 19.96)

Obturator Internus Muscle

Origin

- Inside of the obturator membrane
- Mediocaudal bone rim of the obturator foramen

Insertion

Trochanteric fossa

Action

- Stabilization of the hip joint
- Outward rotation in the hip joint

Innervation

Obturator nerve (L5–S2)

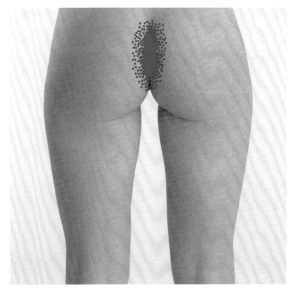

Fig. 19.95

External Anal Sphincter Muscle

Origin

Ring-shaped closing muscle

Insertion

Perianal in subcutaneous, superficial, and deep connective tissue

Action

Closing the anal canal (fecal continence)

Innervation

Pudendal nerve (S2–S4)

Levator Ani Muscle

Origin

- Backside of the pubic bone
- Tendinous arc of the levator ani
- Ischiadic spine

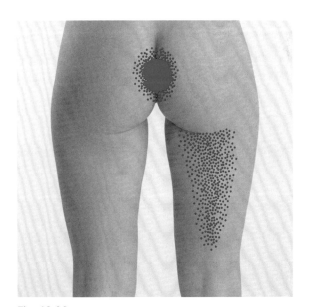

Fig. 19.96

Insertion

- Anococcygeal ligament
- Loop-shaped towards the rectum

Action

- Reinforcement of the pelvic floor
- Maintaining continence

Innervation

Ventral branches of spinal nerves S3–S4

Coccygeus Muscle

Origin

- Sacrospinous ligament
- Ischiadic spine

Insertion

- Anococcygeal ligament
- Coccyx

Action

Reinforcement of the pelvic floor

Innervation

Ventral branches of spinal nerves S4–S5

Trigger Point Location

Trigger points are found by rectal, vaginal, or pelvic floor palpation

Referred Pain

- Coccyx
- Caudal sacrum
- Anal area
- Dorsal thigh (obturator internus)

Associated Internal Organs

- Rectum
- Urinary bladder
- Uterus, adnexa, prostate

▪ Gluteus Maximus Muscle (Figs. 19.97, 19.98)

Origin

- Outside of the wing of the ilium behind the posterior gluteal line
- Posterior third of the iliac crest
- Thoracolumbar fascia
- Sacrum
- Sacrotuberous ligament
- Coccyx

Insertion

- Gluteal tuberosity of the femur
- Iliotibial tract (runs to the lateral condyle of the tibia)

Action

- Extension in the hip joint
- Outward rotation in the hip joint

Innervation

Inferior gluteal nerve (L5–S2)

Trigger Point Location

You achieve good palpation of the trigger points by making the patient lie on the side with the side to be examined facing upward and slightly flexing the legs:

TP1   Approximately at the upper edge of the gluteal fold not far from the insertion of the muscle to the sacrum

TP2   Slightly cranial from the ischiadic tuber

TP3   On the mediocaudal border of the muscle—at the caudal end of the gluteal fold—well palpable with pinching palpation

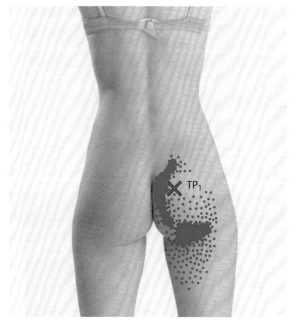

Fig. 19.97

Referred Pain

TP1   From the ISJ along the gluteal fold into the caudal muscle area and the beginning of posterior thigh

TP2   Across the entire muscle with emphasis on the caudal sacrum, the lateral area below the iliac crest, and the caudal buttocks: The pain is partly felt deep down, as if the small gluteus muscles were hurting. No referred pain into the coccyx

TP3   Coccyx and mediocaudal muscle area

Associated Internal Organs

None

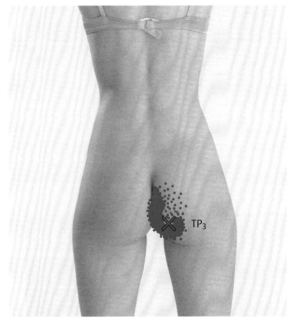

Fig. 19.98

▪ Gluteus Medius Muscle (Figs. 19.99, 19.100, 19.101)

Origin

Outside of the ilium (between the anterior and posterior gluteal line)

Insertion

Greater trochanter (dorsolateral)

Action

- Abduction in the hip joint
- Inward rotation in the hip joint (ventral and lateral part)
- Outward rotation in the hip joint (dorsal and medial part)
- Horizontal stabilization of the pelvis in the swing leg phase of the gait

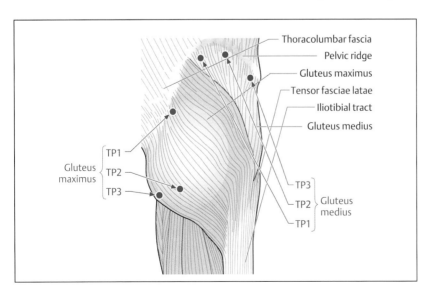

Fig. 19.99

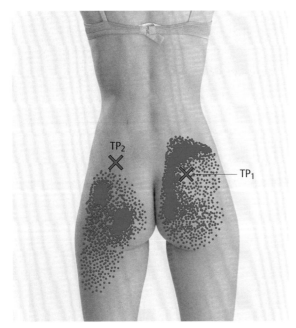

Fig. 19.100

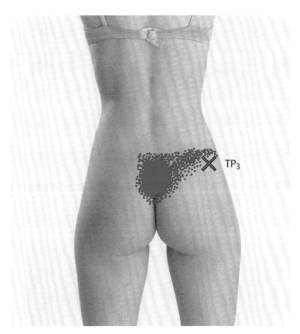

Fig. 19.101

Innervation

Superior gluteal nerve (L4–S1)

Trigger Point Location

Palpate the trigger points in contralateral side position with flexed legs:

TP1   In the posterior muscle belly not far below the iliac crest and in the vicinity of the ISJ

TP2   Immediately below the iliac crest approximately in the center of its course

TP3   It is also found immediately below the iliac crest, but slightly further ventrally in the vicinity of the ASIS

Referred Pain

TP1   The pain radiates from the posterior area of the iliac crest through the ISJ and sacrum into the entire buttocks

TP2   The pain projection runs across the lateral and central gluteal area into the posterior and lateral proximal thigh

TP3   Along the iliac crest and lower lumbar area, the pain radiates especially into the sacrum

Associated Internal Organs

None

■ Gluteus Minimus Muscle (Figs. 19.102, 19.103)

Origin

Outside of the ilium (between the anterior and posterior gluteal lines)

Insertion

Greater trochanter (ventral)

Action

* Abduction in the hip joint
* Inward rotation in the hip joint (ventral and lateral section)
* Horizontal stabilization of the hip in the swing leg phase of the gait

Innervation

Superior gluteal nerve (L4–S1)

Trigger Point Location

* Anterior trigger points: They are found at the height of the ASIS, but slightly further below the iliac crest than in the gluteus medius
* Posterior trigger points: You find these in the entire muscle along the upper edge of its origin

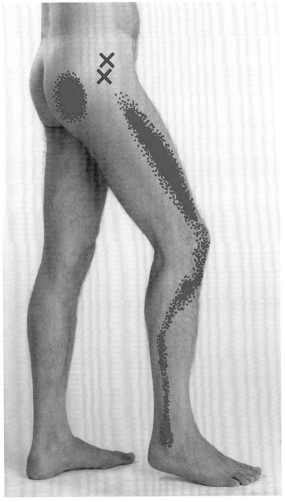

Fig. 19.102

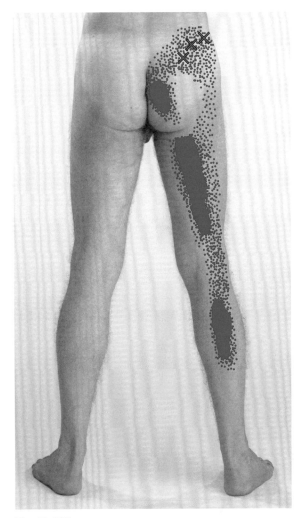

Fig. 19.103

Referred Pain

- Anterior trigger points: Pain is projected into the lower and lateral buttocks, the lateral thigh, knee, and shank
- Posterior trigger points: Throughout the entire buttocks, especially caudal-medial, and continuing on

into the posterior thigh, back of the knee, and proximal third of the shank

Associated Internal Organs

None

■ Piriformis Muscle (Figs. 19.104, 19.105)

Origin

Pelvic side of the sacrum in the area of the anterior sacral foramina 2–4

Insertion

Greater trochanter

Action

- Outward rotation in the hip joint
- Inward rotation in the hip joint at 90° flexed hip
- Abduction in the hip joint at 90° flexed hip

Innervation

Ventral branches of the spinal nerves S1–S2

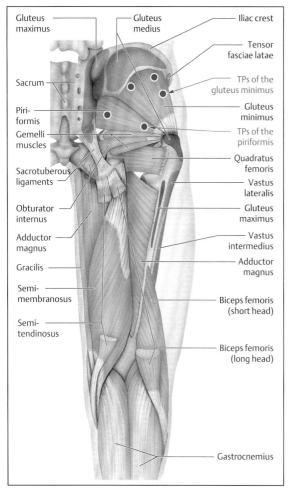

Fig. 19.104

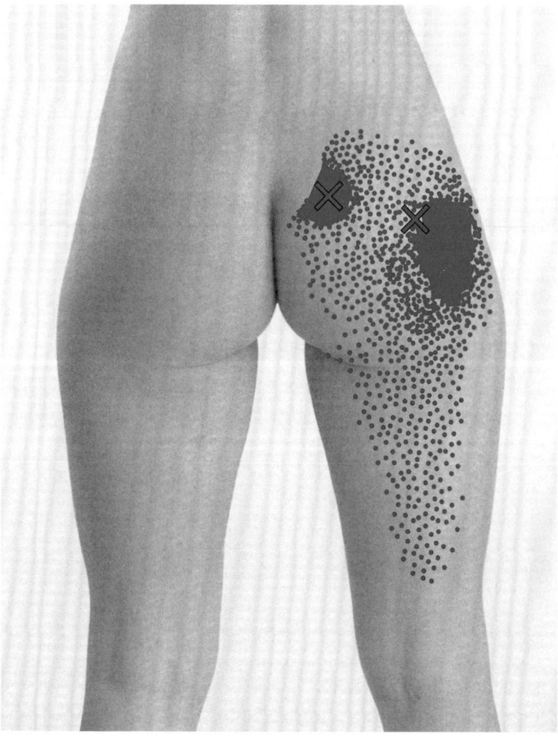

Fig. 19.105

Trigger Point Location

For an auxiliary line for localizing trigger points, connect the proximal end of the greater trochanter to that point of the sacrum that corresponds to the ilium. The upper edge of the piriformis lies approximately on this line:

TP1   When you divide the described auxiliary line into thirds, this trigger point lies slightly lateral to the transition from the middle to the lateral third

TP2   At the medial end of the auxiliary line

Referred Pain

• ISJ
• Entire gluteal area
• Dorsal two-thirds of the thigh

Associated Internal Organs

• Urinary bladder
• Sigmoid colon
• Rectum
• Uterus, ovaries, adnexa, prostate

19.6 Muscles of Hip, Thigh, and Knee Pain

▪ Tensor Fasciae Latae Muscle (Fig. 19.106)

Origin

Iliac crest between the iliac tubercle and the ASIS (outside)

Insertion

Through the iliotibial tract to the front side of the lateral condyle of the tibia

Action

- Abduction in the hip joint
- Stabilizing the knee in extension

Innervation

Superior gluteal nerve (L4–S1)

Trigger Point Location

At the front edge of the muscle in the proximal third

Referred Pain

- Hip joint
- Anterolateral thigh, possibly all the way to the knee

Associated Internal Organs

None

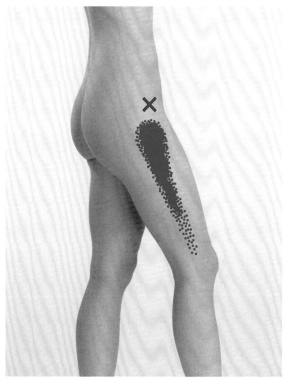

Fig. 19.106

▪ Sartorius Muscle (Figs. 19.107, 19.108)

Origin

Slightly below the ASIS

Insertion

Tibial tuberosity, medial edge

Action

- Flexion in the hip joint
- Abduction in the hip joint
- Outward rotation in the hip joint
- Flexion in the knee joint
- Inward rotation in the knee joint

Innervation

Femoral nerve (L3–L4)

Trigger Point Location

TP1–3 lie in the course of the muscle from proximal to distal.

Referred Pain

Ventral and medial thigh (in the course of the muscle)

Associated Internal Organs

None

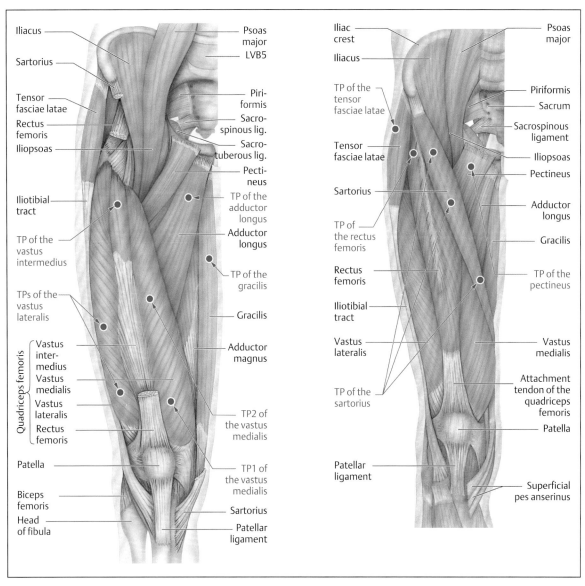

Fig. 19.107

▪ Pectineus Muscle

Origin

- Pecten pubis
- Superior pubic ramus

Insertion

Pectineal line below the greater trochanter

Action

- Flexion in the hip joint
- Adduction in the hip joint
- Inward rotation in the hip joint

Innervation

- Femoral nerve (L2–L3)
- Occasionally also obturator nerve (L2–L3)

Trigger Point Location

Distal of the superior pubic ramus (see **Fig. 19.108**)

Referred Pain

Deep inguinal pain immediately below the inguinal ligament

Associated Internal Organs

- Urinary bladder
- Uterus, adnexa, prostate

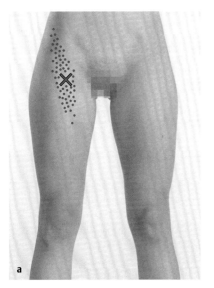
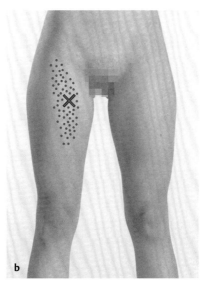
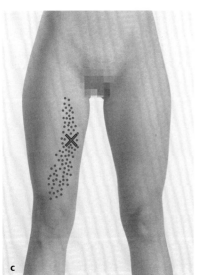
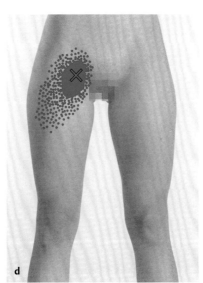

Fig. 19.108a–d

■ Quadriceps Femoris Muscle (Figs. 19.109, 19.110, 19.111)

Rectus Femoris Muscle

Origin

• Anterior inferior iliac spine (AIIS)
• Ilium, cranial to the acetabulum

Vastus Lateralis Muscle

Origin

• Upper section of the intertrochanteric line
• Greater trochanter
• Lateral lip of the linea aspera
• Lateral supracondylar ridge
• Lateral intermuscular septum of the femur

Vastus Medialis Muscle

Origin

• Lower section of the intertrochanteric line
• Medial lip of the linea aspera
• Spiral line
• Medial intermuscular septum of the femur

Vastus Intermedius Muscle

Origin

Frontal and exterior side of the femur (up to about one hand-width above the condyles)

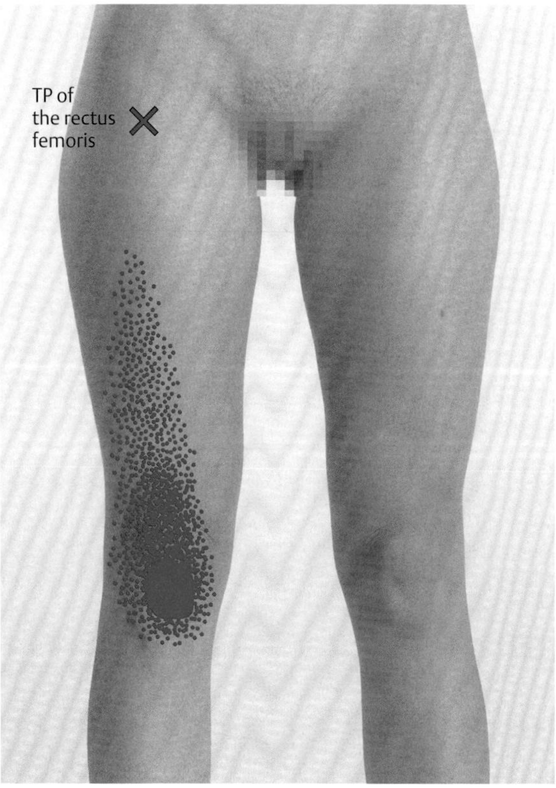

TP of
the rectus
femoris

Fig. 19.109

Rectus Femoris, Vastus Lateralis, Vastus Medialis, and Vastus Intermedius Muscles

Insertion

* Through the quadriceps tendon to the patella
* Through the patellar ligament to the tuberosity of the tibia

Action

* Extension at the knee joint
* Rectus femoris also hip bend

Innervation

Femoral nerve (L3–L4)

Trigger Point Location

* Trigger point of the rectus femoris: Slightly caudal of the AIIS
* Trigger point of the vastus medialis: You find this at the medial rim of the muscle. TP1 lies further distal, slightly above the patella, and TP2 almost exactly in the middle of the thigh
* Trigger point of the vastus intermedius: Trigger points are difficult to palpate because a digital examination is difficult due to the deep-lying position of this muscle. The trigger points lie proximal in the muscle belly, but more distal than the trigger points of the rectus femoris. Access to these trigger points is obtained by proximal palpation of the lateral rim of the rectus femoris and from there palpating deeply into the thigh
* Trigger point of the vastus lateralis: Due to its deep position in the thigh, palpation of its trigger points is very difficult. They are distributed throughout the entire muscle belly and manifest with typical referred pain only when the muscle is compressed onto the femur. (See also **Fig. 19.107**)

Referred Pain

Trigger point of the rectus femoris:
* Knee joint
* Around the patella
* Medial thigh

Trigger point of the vastus medialis: ventromedial knee (TP1) and thigh (TP2) area.

Trigger point of the vastus intermedius: in the entire ventral thigh, concentrated in the middle of the thigh.

Trigger points of the vastus lateralis: lateral thigh and knee area.

Associated Internal Organs

None

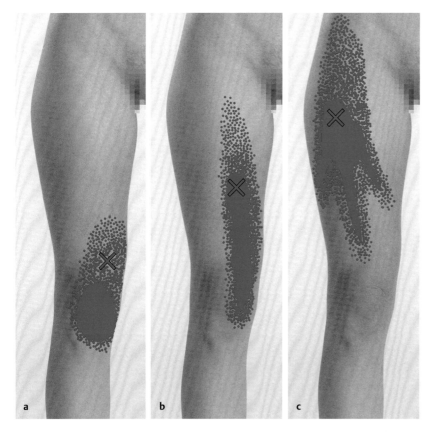

Fig. 19.110a–c

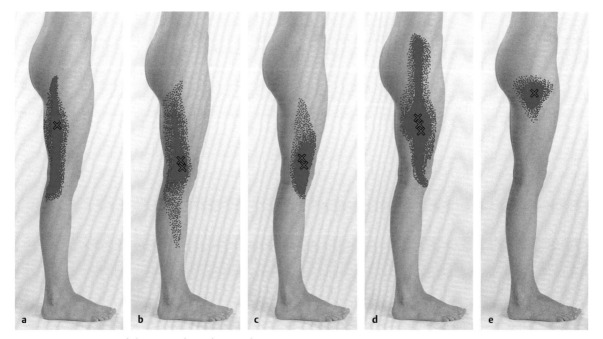

Fig. 19.111a–e TPs of the vastus lateralis muscle

■ Gracilis and Adductor Longus, Brevis, and Magnus Muscles

Gracilis Muscle (Fig. 19.112)

Origin

Inferior pubic ramus (outside)

Insertion

Front side of the tibia (below the sartorius)

Action

- Adduction in the hip joint
- Flexion in the knee joint
- Inward rotation in the knee joint (when knee is flexed)

Innervation

Obturator nerve (L2–L3)

Trigger Point Location

In the middle third of the muscle belly

Referred Pain

Inside of the thigh

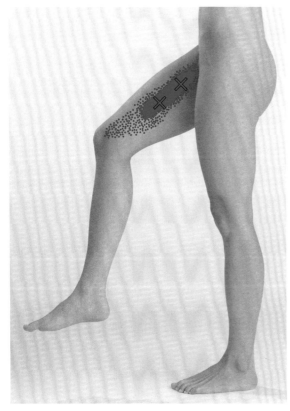

Fig. 19.112

Associated Internal Organs

- Uterus, adnexa
- Prostate
- Urinary bladder

Adductor Longus Muscle

Origin

- Shaft of the pubic bone
- Pubic tubercle (underneath and medial)

Insertion

Medial lip of the linea aspera (distal two-thirds)

Action

- Adduction in the hip joint
- Inward rotation in the hip joint

Innervation

Obturator nerve (L2–L3)

Adductor Brevis Muscle (Fig. 19.113)

Origin

Inferior ramus and shaft of the pubic bone

Insertion

Linea aspera (proximal third)

Action

Adduction in the hip joint

Innervation

Obturator nerve (L2–L3)

Trigger Point Location

You can palpate the trigger points well when you pre-tense the muscles by flexing and abducting the hip. For this purpose, the patient lies in supine position. The trigger points lied in the proximal half of the muscles.

Referred Pain

- Groin
- Ventromedial thigh
- Suprapatellar
- Along the rim of the tibia

Associated Internal Organs

- Uterus, adnexa
- Prostate
- Testicles
- Urinary bladder

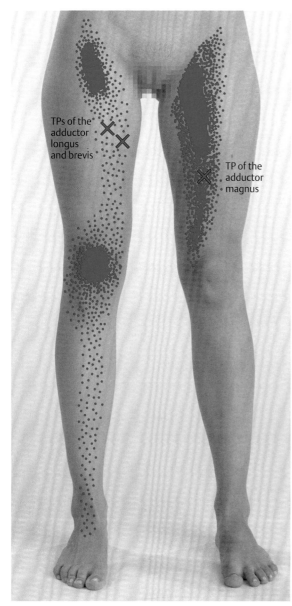

TPs of the adductor longus and brevis

TP of the adductor magnus

Fig. 19.113

Adductor Magnus Muscle (Fig. 19.114)

Origin

- Ramus of the ischium
- Inferior ramus of the pubis
- Ischiadic tuber

Insertion

- Linea aspera up to the gluteal tuberosity
- Adductor tubercle of the femur

Action

- Extension in the hip joint
- Adduction in the hip joint
- Inward rotation in the hip joint

Innervation

- Obturator nerve (L2–L4)
- Tibial nerve (L4–S3)

Trigger Point Location

TP1 In the middle of the muscle, near the insertion of the linea aspera

TP2 Near the origin at the ischium and pubis (see **Fig. 19.113**)

Referred Pain

TP1 Groin and ventromedial thigh, not all the way down to the knee

TP2 Pubic bone, vagina, rectum, bladder, or other diffuse pain in the small pelvis

Associated Internal Organs

- Uterus, adnexa
- Prostate
- Urinary bladder

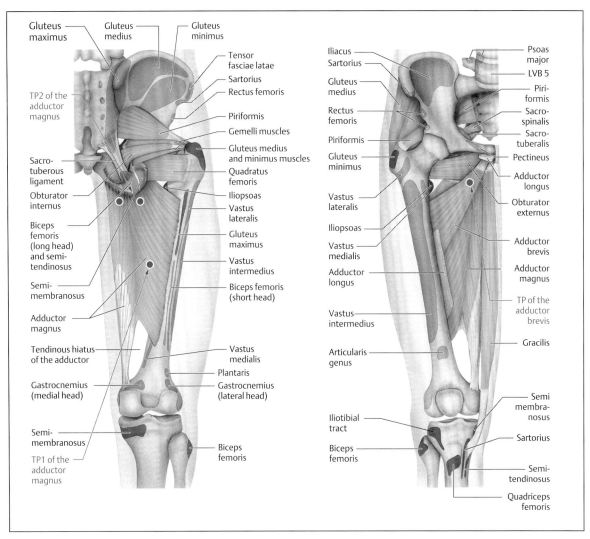

Fig. 19.114

■ Biceps Femoris, Semitendinosus, and Semimembranosus Muscles

Biceps Femoris Muscle (Fig. 19.115)

Origin

- Ischiadic tuber (backside)
- Lateral lip of the linea aspera (middle third)

Insertion

- Apex of head of fibula
- Lateral supracondylar line of the femur
- Lateral collateral ligament
- Lateral condyle of the tibia

Action

- Extension in the hip joint
- Flexion in the knee joint
- Outward rotation in the knee joint

Innervation

Tibial and fibular nerve (L4–S3)

Trigger Point Location

Several trigger points are found in the middle third of the posterolateral thigh.

Referred Pain

- Back of the knee (primary pain)
- Proximal posterolateral lower leg
- Posterolateral thigh, not up to the gluteal fold

Associated Internal Organs

None

Semitendinosus Muscle (Fig. 19.116)

Origin

Ischiadic tuber (backside)

Insertion

Medial surface of the tibia (below the gracilis)

Action

- Extension in the hip joint
- Flexion in the knee joint
- Inward rotation in the knee joint

Innervation

Tibial nerve (L5–S1)

Semimembranosus Muscle
(Fig. 19.116)

Origin

Ischiadic tuber (backside)

Insertion

- Medial condyle of the tibia
- Oblique popliteal ligament
- Fascia of the popliteus

Action

- Extension in the hip joint
- Flexion in the knee joint
- Inward rotation in the knee joint

Innervation

Tibial nerve (L5–S1)

Trigger Point Location

Several trigger points are found in the middle third of the posteromedial thigh.

Referred Pain

- Caudal end of the buttocks and gluteal fold (primary pain)
- Posteromedial thigh
- Medial half of the back of the knee and of the calf

Associated Internal Organs

None

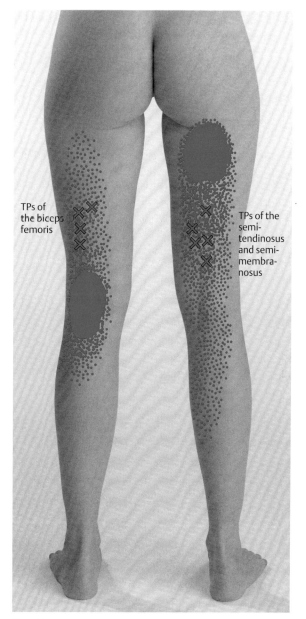

TPs of the biceps femoris

TPs of the semi-tendinosus and semi-membra-nosus

Fig. 19.115

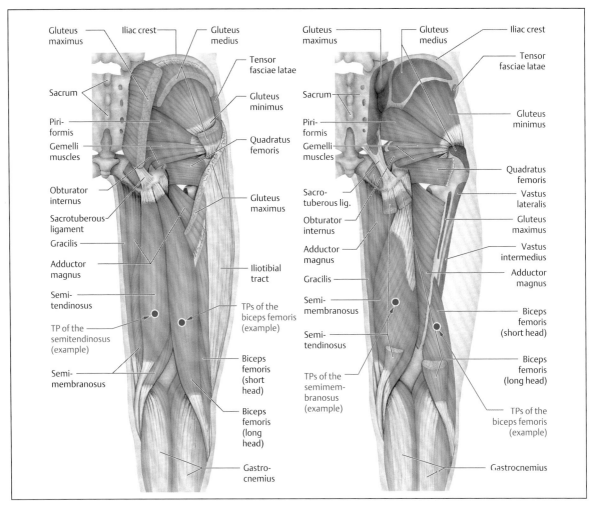

Fig. 19.116

▪ Popliteus Muscle (Figs. 19.117, 19.118)

Origin

Posterior side of the tibia (above the line for the soleus muscle and below the tibial condyles)

Insertion

- Lateral epicondyle of the femur
- Radiating into the knee joint capsule
- Connection to the lateral meniscus (posterior horn)

Action

- Inward rotation in the knee joint
- Pulls the lateral meniscus backward

Innervation

Tibial nerve (L5–S1)

Trigger Point Location

In the proximal half of the origin of the muscle, near the tibia

Referred Pain

Knee joint

Associated Internal Organs

None

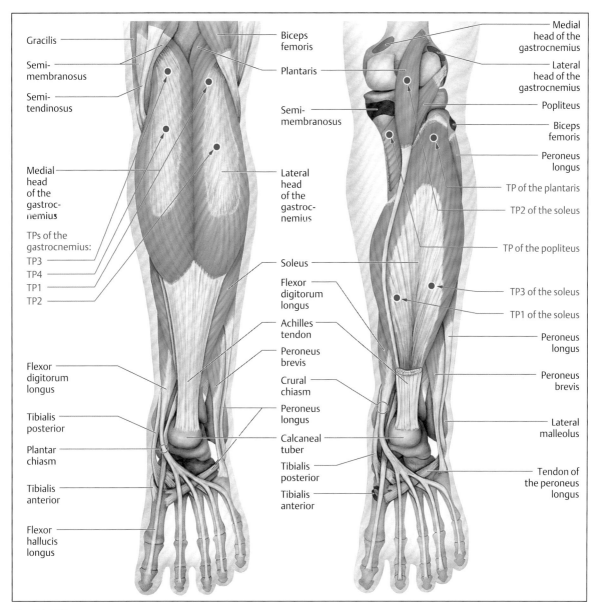

Fig. 19.117

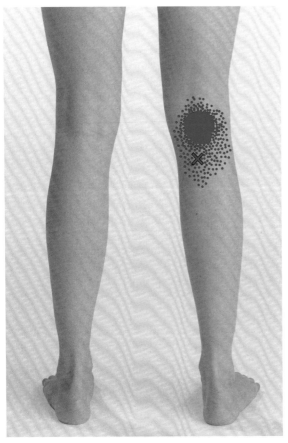

Fig. 19.118

19.7   Muscles of Lower Leg, Ankle, and Foot Pain

▪ Tibialis Anterior Muscle (Figs. 19.119, 19.120)

Origin

- Lateral side of the tibia (proximal half)
- Interosseous membrane

Insertion

- Medial cuneiform bone (plantar side)
- Base of the metatarsal bone I

Action

- Dorsal extension
- Inversion of the foot
- Stabilization of the longitudinal arch of the foot

Innervation

Deep fibular nerve (L4–L5)

Trigger Point Location

In the upper third of the muscle belly (transition from the proximal to the middle third of the lower leg)

Referred Pain

- Ventromedial area of the upper ankle joint
- Dorsal and medial at the big toe
- A narrow band from the trigger point anteromedial through the lower leg to the big toe

Associated Internal Organs

None

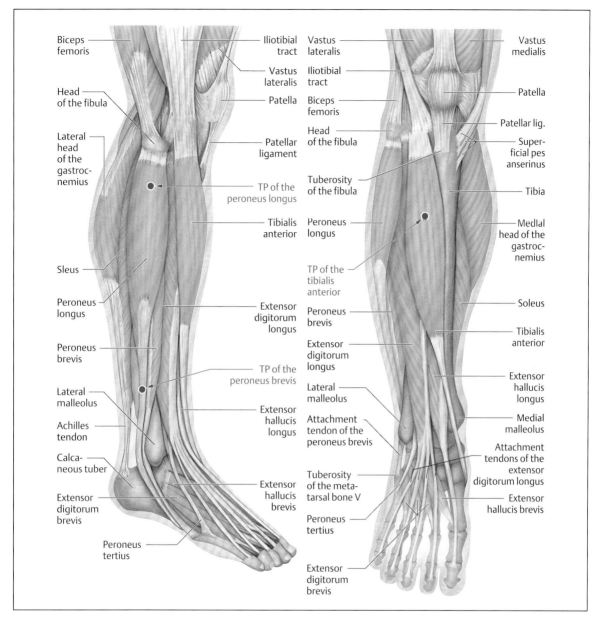

Fig. 19.119

▪ Tibialis Posterior Muscle (Figs. 19.121, 19.122)

Origin

Backside of the tibia and fibula (between the medial crest, interosseous border, and interosseous membrane)

Insertion

- Tuberosity of the navicular bone
- All tarsal bones (excepting the talus)
- Medial tarsal ligaments (e.g., deltoid ligament)

Action

- Plantar flexion
- Inversion of the foot
- Stabilization of the longitudinal arch of the foot

Innervation

Tibial nerve (L4–L5)

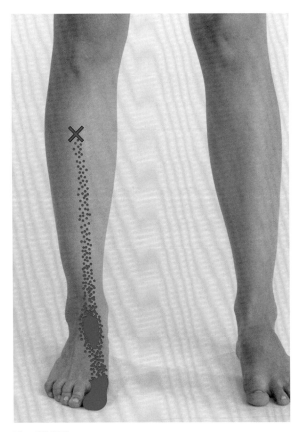

Fig. 19.120

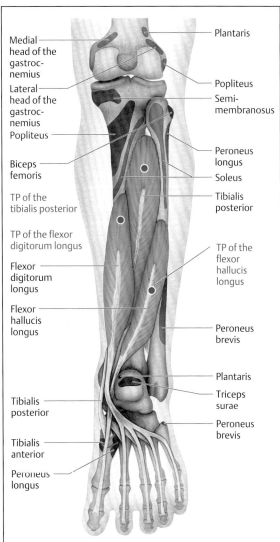

Medial head of the gastrocnemius

Lateral head of the gastrocnemius

Popliteus

Biceps femoris

TP of the tibialis posterior

TP of the flexor digitorum longus

Flexor digitorum longus

Flexor hallucis longus

Tibialis posterior

Tibialis anterior

Peroneus longus

Plantaris

Popliteus

Semi-membranosus

Peroneus longus

Soleus

Tibialis posterior

TP of the flexor hallucis longus

Peroneus brevis

Plantaris

Triceps surae

Peroneus brevis

Fig. 19.121

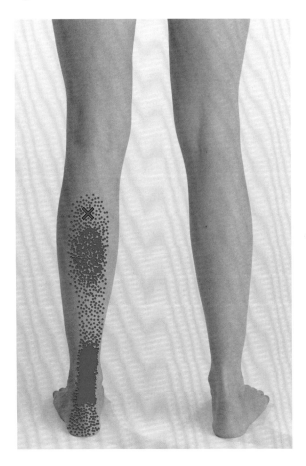

Fig. 19.122

Trigger Point Location

Lateral to the posterior rim of the tibia and in the proximal quarter of the interosseous membrane. It can only be palpated through the soleus.

Referred Pain

• Achilles tendon (primary pain)

• From the trigger point caudal into the middle of the lower leg through the heel and sole referring to toes 1–5

Associated Internal Organs

None

▪ Peroneus Longus, Brevis, and Tertius Muscles

Peroneus Longus Muscle

Origin

• Lateral fascia of the tibia (proximal two-thirds)
• Head of the fibula
• Tibiofibular articulation

Insertion

• Base of the metatarsal bone I
• Medial cuneiform bone

Action

• Plantar flexion
• Eversion of the foot
• Stabilization of the transverse arch of the foot

Innervation

Superficial fibular nerve (L5–S1)

Peroneus Brevis Muscle (Fig. 19.123)

Origin

Lateral fascia of the tibia (distal two-thirds)

Insertion

Tuberosity of the metatarsal bone V

Action

• Dorsal flexion
• Eversion of the foot
• Stabilization of the transverse arch of the foot

Innervation

Superficial fibular nerve (L5–S1)

Trigger Point Location

• Trigger point of the peroneus longus: 2–4 cm distal from the fibula head above the fibula shaft
• Trigger point of the peroneus brevis: at the border between the middle and distal thirds of the lower leg, on both sides of the tendon of the peroneus longus

Referred Pain

• Lateral malleolus, also cranial, caudal, and posterior thereof
• Middle third of the lateral lower leg
• Lateral on the foot

Associated Internal Organs

None

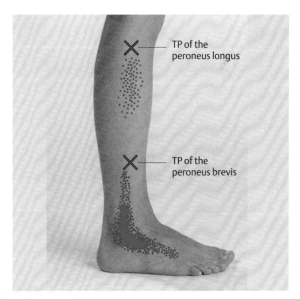

Fig. 19.123

Peroneus Tertius Muscle (Fig. 19.124)

Origin

Anterior border of the fibula (distal third)

Insertion

Metatarsal bone V

Action

- Dorsal flexion
- Eversion of the foot

Innervation

Deep fibular nerve (L5–S1)

Trigger Point Location

Slightly distal and anterior from the peroneus brevis trigger point (see also **Fig. 19.119**)

Referred Pain

- Ventrolateral on the upper ankle joint and on the back of the foot
- Posterior from the lateral malleolus running towards the lateral heel

Associated Internal Organs

None

Gastrocnemius Muscle
(Figs. 19.125, 19.126)

Origin

Medial and lateral condyle of the femur

Insertion

Calcaneal tuber (above the Achilles tendon)

Action

- Plantar flexion
- Knee flexion

Innervation

Tibial nerve (S1–S2)

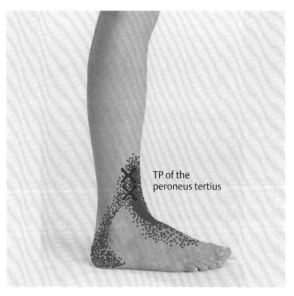

TP of the peroneus tertius

Fig. 19.124

Trigger Point Location

TP1 and TP2   About proximal to the middle of the muscle bellies, one trigger point each in the medial and lateral head of the gastrocnemius

TP3 and TP4   In the medial and lateral heads of the gastrocnemius, in the vicinity of the condyles (see also **Fig. 19.117**)

Referred Pain

TP1   Medial on the sole of the foot
Posteromedial lower leg
Back of the knee and partly up the posterior thigh

TP2–TP4   The referred pain of these three trigger points can be found locally around each trigger point.

Associated Internal Organs

None

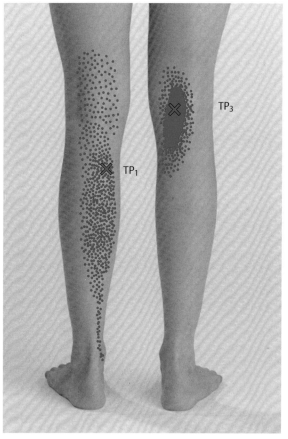

Fig. 19.125

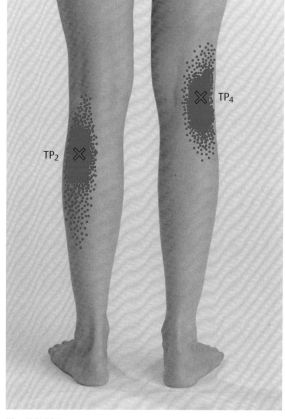

Fig. 19.126

◾ Soleus and Plantaris Muscles (Fig. 19.127)

Soleus Muscle

Origin

- Line of the soleus
- Posterior fascia of the tibia (middle third)
- Neck and posterior fascia of the fibula (proximal third)

Insertion

Calcaneal tuber (above the Achilles tendon)

Action

Plantar flexion

Innervation

Tibial nerve (S1–S2)

Trigger Point Location

TP1   2–3 cm distal from the gastrocnemius heads and slightly medial from the center line
TP2   Near the fibula head (lateral on the calf)
TP3   Further proximal than TP1 and lateral from the center line

Referred Pain

TP1   Achilles tendon
      Heel posterior and plantar
      Sole of the foot
      Slightly proximal to the trigger point
TP2   Upper half of the calf
TP3   ISJ ipsilateral

Associated Internal Organs

None

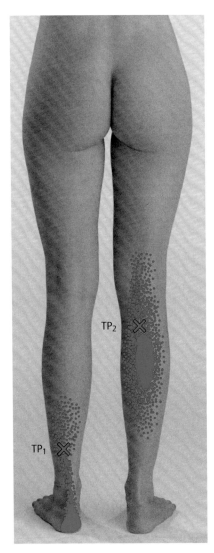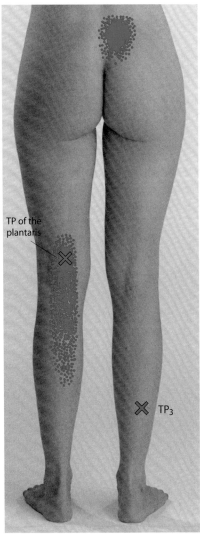

Fig. 19.127

Plantaris Muscle

Origin

Lateral epicondyle of the femur (proximal to the gastrocnemius head)

Insertion

Achilles tendon (medial, below the tendon of the gastrocnemius)

Action

• Plantar flexion
• Knee flexion

Innervation

Tibial nerve (S1–S2)

Trigger Point Location

In the middle of the back of the knee

Referred Pain

Back of the knee and calf up to about the middle of the lower leg

Associated Internal Organs

None

▪ Extensor Digitorum Longus and Hallucis Longus Muscles

(Figs. 19.128, 19.129)

Extensor Digitorum Longus Muscle

Origin

- Fibula (ventral proximal two-thirds)
- Interosseous membrane
- Tibiofibular articulation

Insertion

Dorsal aponeurosis of toes 2–5

Action

Dorsal extension of the toes and foot

Innervation

Deep fibular nerve (L5–S1)

Trigger Point Location

Ca. 8 cm distal from the fibula head between the peroneus longus and tibialis anterior

Referred Pain

- Back of the foot, including toes 2–4
- Ventral lower leg (caudal half)

Associated Internal Organs

None

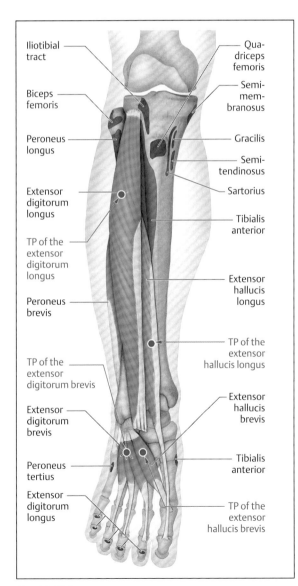

Fig. 19.128

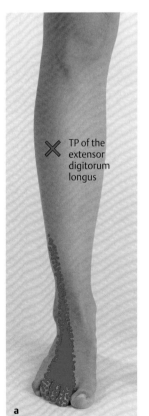
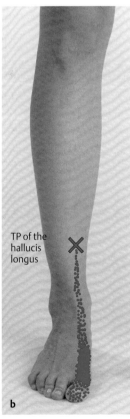

Fig. 19.129

Extensor Hallucis Longus Muscle

Origin

Fibula (middle frontal area)

Insertion

Base of the end phalanx of the big toe

Action

- Dorsal extension of the big toe and foot
- Inversion of the foot

Innervation

Deep peroneal nerve (L5–S1)

Trigger Point Location

Slightly distal from the transition between the middle and caudal third of the lower leg and ventral to the fibula. It lies between the extensor digitorum longus and the tibialis anterior

Referred Pain

Back of the foot in the area of the first metatarsal bone and the big toe, sometimes referring in a small band to the trigger point

Associated Internal Organs

None

▪ Flexor Digitorum Longus and Hallucis Longus Muscles

(Fig. 19.121, Figs. 19.130, 19.131, 19.132, 19.133)

Flexor Digitorum Longus Muscle

Origin

- Posterior fascia of the tibia (distal to the line of the soleus)
- Fibula (above the tendinous arch)

Insertion

Base of the end phalanges of toes 2–5

Action

- Flexion of the toe end joints
- Plantar flexion
- Stabilization of the longitudinal arch of the foot

Innervation

Tibial nerve (S1–S2)

Trigger Point Location

By displacing the medial gastrocnemius belly, you can find the trigger point on the posterior side of the tibia in the proximal third of the medial calf area

Referred Pain

- Sole of the foot (mediolateral) up to toes 2–5 (primary pain)
- Medial malleolus and medial calf area up to the trigger point

Associated Internal Organs

None

Flexor Hallucis Longus Muscle

Origin

- Posterior fascia of the fibula (distal two-thirds)
- Intermuscular septum
- Aponeurosis of the flexor digitorum longus

Insertion

- Base of the proximal phalanx of the big toe
- Fibers to the two medial tendons of the flexor digitorum longus

Action

- Flexion of the base phalanx of the big toe
- Plantar flexion
- Stabilization of the longitudinal arch of the foot

Innervation

Tibial nerve (S2–S3)

Trigger Point Location

At the transition from the middle to the caudal third of the lower leg and slightly lateral to the center line on the dorsal side of the fibula. Palpate it through the superficial calf musculature

Referred Pain

Plantar side of the big toe and metatarsal bone I

Associated Internal Organs

None

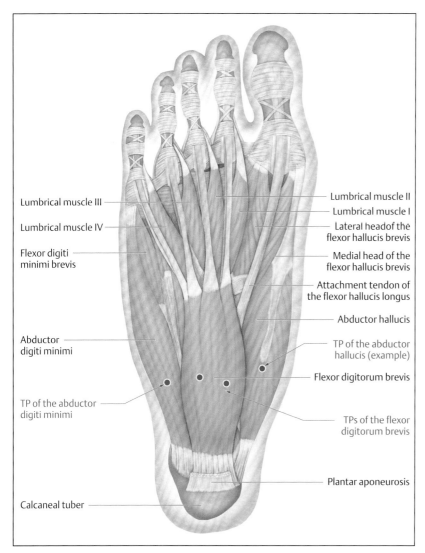

Lumbrical muscle III

Lumbrical muscle IV

Flexor digiti
minimi brevis

Abductor
digiti minimi

TP of the abductor
digiti minimi

Calcaneal tuber

Lumbrical muscle II

Lumbrical muscle I

Lateral head of the
flexor hallucis brevis

Medial head of the
flexor hallucis brevis

Attachment tendon of
the flexor hallucis longus

Abductor hallucis

TP of the abductor
hallucis (example)

Flexor digitorum brevis

TPs of the flexor
digitorum brevis

Plantar aponeurosis

Fig. 19.130

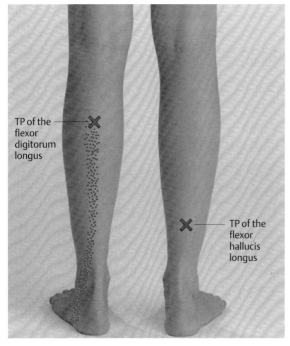

TP of the
flexor
digitorum
longus

TP of the
flexor
hallucis
longus

Fig. 19.131

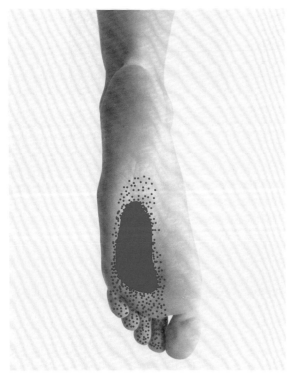

Fig. 19.132

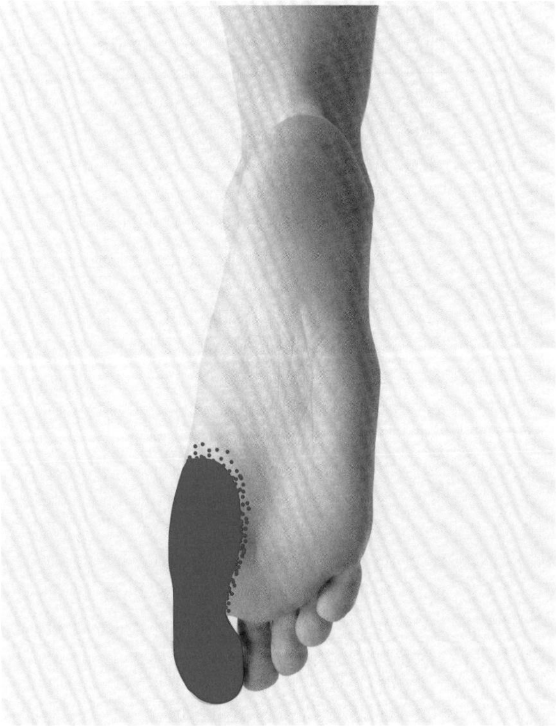

Fig. 19.133

■ Superficial Intrinsic Foot Musculature

Extensor Digitorum Brevis Muscle (Fig. 19.134)

Origin

Calcaneus (dorsal side)

Insertion

• Proximal phalanx of the big toe
• Toes 2–4 (through the long stretch tendons)

Action

Toe extensor

Innervation

Deep fibular nerve (L5–S1)

Trigger Point Location

In the first third of the muscle bellies

Referred Pain

Area on the medial back of the foot near the ankle joint

Associated Internal Organs

None

Extensor Hallucis Brevis Muscle (Fig. 19.134)

Origin

Dorsal side of the calcaneus

Insertion

• Dorsal aponeurosis of the big toe
• Base of the proximal phalanx of the big toe

Action

Dorsal extension in the proximal joint of the big toe

Innervation

Deep fibular nerve (L5–S1)

Trigger Point Location

In the first third of the muscle belly (see also **Fig. 19.128**)

Referred Pain

Area of the medial back of the foot near the ankle joint

Associated Internal Organs

None

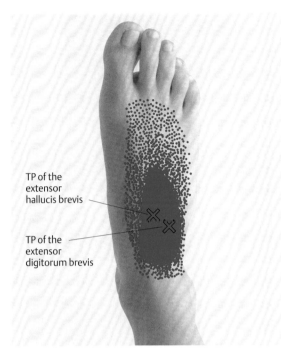

TP of the
extensor
hallucis brevis

TP of the
extensor
digitorum brevis

Fig. 19.134

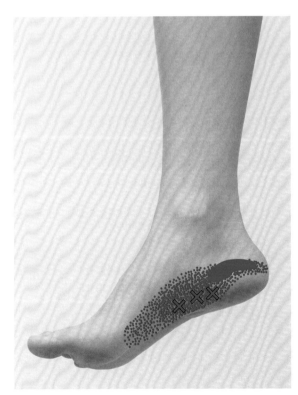

Fig. 19.135

Abductor Hallucis Muscle (Figs. 19.130, 19.135)

Origin

- Medial process of the calcaneal tuber
- Flexor retinaculum

Insertion

Proximal phalanx of the big toe (medial)

Action

- Abduction of the big toe
- Plantar flexion

Innervation

Medial plantar nerve (S1–S2)

Trigger Point Location

Distributed in the muscle belly along the inside edge of the foot

Referred Pain

Inside of the heel and inside edge of the foot

Associated Internal Organs

None

Flexor Digitorum Brevis Muscle (Figs. 19.130, 19.136)

Origin

Calcaneal tuber (plantar)

Insertion

Middle phalanges of toes 2–5 (split tendons)

Action

- Flexion of toes 2–5
- Stabilization of the arch of the foot

Innervation

Medial plantar nerve (S1–S2)

Trigger Point Location

In the muscle belly in the proximal middle area of the sole of the foot

Referred Pain

Metatarsal heads II–IV with only slight tendency to radiate further

Associated Internal Organs

None

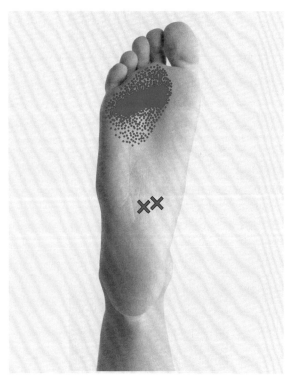

Fig. 19.136

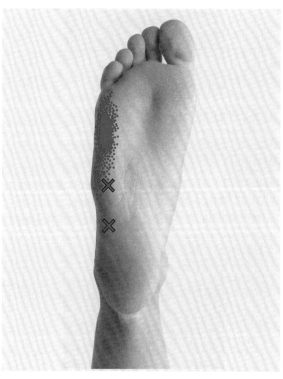

Fig. 19.137

Abductor Digiti Minimi Muscle
(Figs. 19.130, 19.138)

Origin

Medial and lateral processes of the calcaneal tuber

Insertion

- Base of the proximal phalanx of toe 5 (lateral)
- Metatarsal bone V

Action

- Flexion of toe 5
- Abduction of toe 5
- Stabilization of the longitudinal arch of the foot

Innervation

Lateral plantar nerve (S2–S3)

Trigger Point Location

Distributed throughout the muscle belly along the outer edge of the sole of the foot

Referred Pain

Metatarsal head V with only slight tendency to radiate into the area of the lateral sole of the foot

Associated Internal Organs

None

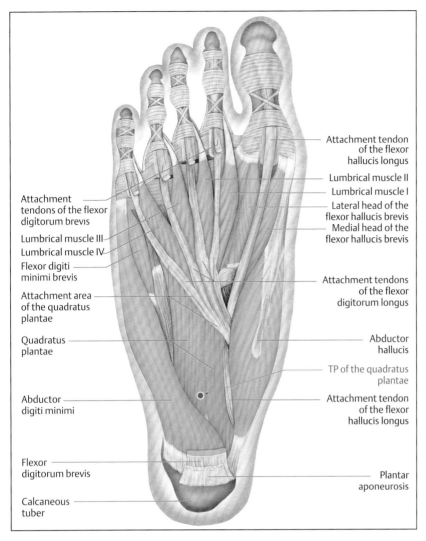

Attachment tendon
of the flexor
hallucis longus

Lumbrical muscle II
Lumbrical muscle I
Lateral head of the
flexor hallucis brevis
Medial head of the
flexor hallucis brevis

Attachment tendons
of the flexor
digitorum longus

Abductor
hallucis

TP of the quadratus
plantae

Attachment tendon
of the flexor
hallucis longus

Plantar
aponeurosis

Attachment
tendons of the flexor
digitorum brevis

Lumbrical muscle III
Lumbrical muscle IV
Flexor digiti
minimi brevis

Attachment area
of the quadratus
plantae

Quadratus
plantae

Abductor
digiti minimi

Flexor
digitorum brevis

Calcaneous
tuber

Fig. 19.138

▪ Deep Intrinsic Foot Musculature

Quadratus Plantae Muscle
(Figs. 19.139, 19.140, 19.141)

Origin

Dual-headed from the edges of the calcaneus

Insertion

Tendon of the flexor digitorum longus

Action

Assists in the flexion of toes 2–5

Innervation

Lateral plantar nerve (S2–S3)

Trigger Point Location

Can be palpated immediately in front of the heel through the plantar aponeurosis

Referred Pain

Plantar side of the heel

Associated Internal Organs

None

Dorsal Interossei Muscles

Origin

Dual-headed from the insides of all metatarsal bones

Insertion

- Base of the proximal phalanges (toe 2: medial side, toes 2–4, lateral side)
- Dorsal aponeurosis of the toes

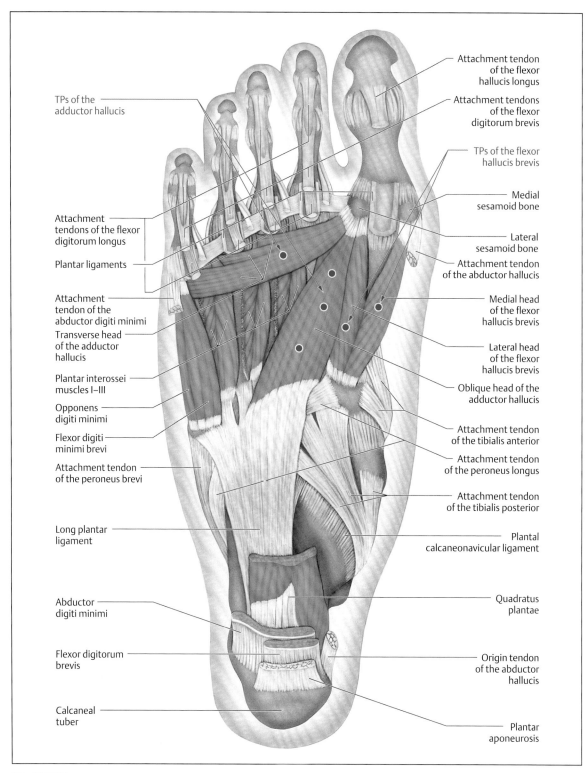

TPs of the adductor hallucis

Attachment tendons of the flexor digitorum longus

Plantar ligaments

Attachment tendon of the abductor digiti minimi

Transverse head of the adductor hallucis

Plantar interossei muscles I–III

Opponens digiti minimi

Flexor digiti minimi brevi

Attachment tendon of the peroneus brevi

Long plantar ligament

Abductor digiti minimi

Flexor digitorum brevis

Calcaneal tuber

Attachment tendon of the flexor hallucis longus

Attachment tendons of the flexor digitorum brevis

TPs of the flexor hallucis brevis

Medial sesamoid bone

Lateral sesamoid bone

Attachment tendon of the abductor hallucis

Medial head of the flexor hallucis brevis

Lateral head of the flexor hallucis brevis

Oblique head of the adductor hallucis

Attachment tendon of the tibialis anterior

Attachment tendon of the peroneus longus

Attachment tendon of the tibialis posterior

Plantal calcaneonavicular ligament

Quadratus plantae

Origin tendon of the abductor hallucis

Plantar aponeurosis

Fig. 19.139

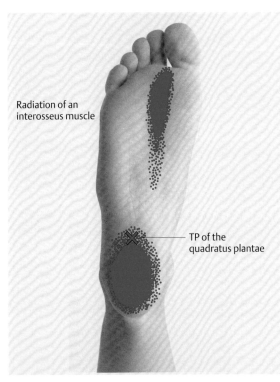

Radiation of an
interosseus muscle

TP of the
quadratus plantae

Fig. 19.140

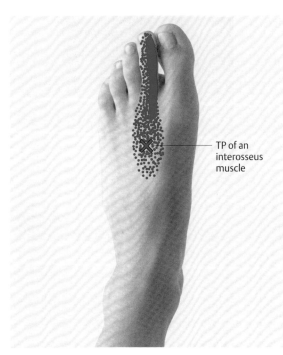

TP of an
interosseus
muscle

Fig. 19.141

Action

Abduction of toes 2–4

Innervation

Lateral plantar nerve (S2–S3)

Plantar Interossei Muscles

Origin

One-headed from the metatarsal bones III–V

Insertion

- Base of the proximal phalanges of toes 3–5
- Dorsal aponeurosis of the toes

Action

Adduction of toes 3–5

Innervation

Lateral plantar nerve (S2–S3)

Trigger Point Location

Between the metatarsal bones. Palpate from plantar and dorsal

Referred Pain

The referred pain of these trigger points is found along that side of the toes at which the tendon of the muscle is inserted. The pain can project to dorsal as well as to plantar

Associated Internal Organs

None

Adductor Hallucis Muscle (Fig. 19.142)

Origin

- Oblique head: base of the metatarsal bones II–IV
- Transverse head: capsule ligaments of the proximal joints of toes 3–5 and transverse deep metatarsal ligament

Insertion

- Lateral sesamoid bone
- Proximal phalanx of the big toe (lateral)

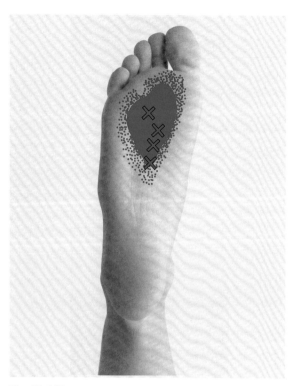

Fig. 19.142

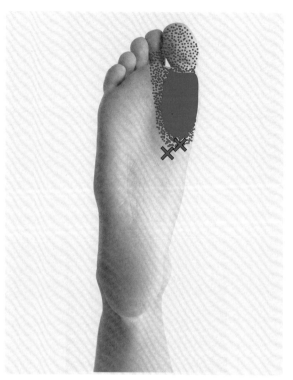

Fig. 19.143

Action

- Adduction of the big toe
- Flexion of the big toe
- Stabilization of the arch of the foot

Innervation

Lateral plantar nerve (S2–S3)

Trigger Point Location

Palpable in the area of the metatarsal heads I–IV through the aponeurosis

Referred Pain

In an area around the metatarsal heads II–IV

Associated Internal Organs

None

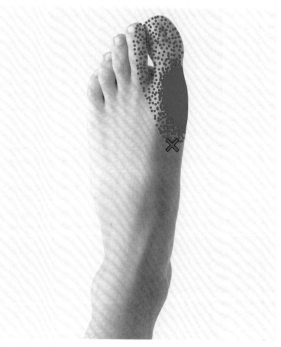

Fig. 19.144

Flexor Hallucis Brevis Muscle
(Figs. 19.143, 19.144)

Origin

- Cuboid bone
- Cuneiform bones 1–3

Insertion

Base of the proximal joint of the big toe (running with one tendon each lateral and medial across the sesamoid bones)

Action

- Flexion of the big toe
- Stabilization of the arch of the foot

Innervation

Tibial nerve (S2–S3)

Trigger Point Location

At the medial inner edge of the foot roughly proximal to the metatarsal head I

Referred Pain

Plantar and medial around the metatarsal head I and including toes 1 and 2

Associated Internal Organs

None

Bibliography

Muscle Chains (Richter)

[1] Ahonen J, Lathinen T, Sandström M, Pogliani G, Wirhed R. *Sportmedizin und Trainingslehre*. Stuttgart: Schattauer; 1999

[2] American Academy of Osteopathy. *52 AAO Yearbooks from 1938–1998*. Indianapolis, AAO; 2001

[3] Amigues J. *Osteopathie-Kompendium*. Stuttgart: Sonntag; 2004

[4] Arbuckle BG. *The Selected Writings*. Indianapolis: AAO; 1994

[5] Barral J. *Manipulations Uro-genitales*. Paris: Maloine; 1984

[6] Barral J. *Le Thorax*. Paris: Maloine; 1989

[7] Barral JP, Croibier A. *Trauma. Ein osteopathischer Ansatz*. Kötzting: Verlag f. Ganzheitl. Med.; 2003

[8] Becker RE. *Life in Motion*. Fort Worth: Stillness Press; 1997

[9] Becker RE. *The Stillness of Life*. Fort Worth: Stillness Press; 2000

[10] Beckers D, Deckers J. *Ganganalyse und Gangschulung*. Berlin: Springer; 1997

[11] Benichou A. *Os Clés, Os Suspendus*. Paris: SPEK; 2001

[12] van den Berg F. *Angewandte Physiologie*. Stuttgart: Thieme; 2002

[13] Bobath B. *Hémiplegie de l'Adulte Bilans et Traitement*. Paris: Masson; 1978

[14] Bogduk N. *Klinische Anatomie von Lendenwirbelsäule und Sakrum*. Berlin: Springer 2000

[15] Boland U. *Logiques de Pathologies Orthopédiques en Chaînes Ascendantes & Descendantes et la Méthode Exploratoire des "Delta Pondéral."* Paris: Frison-Roche; 1996

[16] Bouchet A, Cuilleret J. *Anatomie, Vols I–IV*. Paris: SIMEP; 1983

[17] Bourdiol RJ. *Pied et Statique*. Paris: Maisonneuve; 1980

[18] Bricot B. *La Reprogrammation Posturale Globale*. Montpellier: Sauramps Medical; 1996

[19] Brokmeier A. *Manuelle Therapie*. 3rd ed. Stuttgart: Hippokrates; 2001

[20] Brügger A. *Die Erkrankungen des Bewegungsapparates und seines Nervensystems*. Stuttgart: G. Fischer; 1997

[21] Buck M, Beckers D, Adler SS. *PNF in der Praxis*. Berlin: Springer; 2001

[22] Buekens J. *Osteopathische Diagnose und Behandlung*. Stuttgart: Hippokrates; 1997

[23] van Buskirk RL. *The Still Technique*. Indianapolis: AAO; 2000

[24] Busquet L, Gabarel B. *Ophtalmologie et Ostéopathie*. Paris: Maloine; 1988

[25] Busquet L. *Les Chaînes Musculaires, Vol I. Du Tronc et de la Colonne Cervicale*. 2nd ed. Paris: Maloine; 1985

[26] Busquet L. *Les Chaînes Musculaires, Vol II. Lordose-cyphoses-scolioses et Déformations Thoraciques*. Paris: Frison-Roche; 1992

[27] Busquet L. *Les Chaînes Musculaires, Vol III. La Pubalgie*. Paris: Frison-Roche; 1993

[28] Busquet L. *Les Chaînes Musculaires, Vol IV. Membres Inférieurs*. Paris: Frison-Roche; 1995

[29] Busquet L. *Les Chaînes Musculaires, Vol V. Traitement Crâne*. Paris: Frison-Roche; 2004

[29a] Busquet L. *L'Osteopathie Cranienne*. Paris: Maloine; 1985

[30] Busquet-Vanderheyden M. (editor Busquet L): *Les Chaînes Musculaires, Vol. VI. La Chaîne Viscérale*. Paris: Editions Busquet; 2004

[31] Butler DS. *Rehabilitation und Prävention*. Berlin: Springer; 1998

[32] Calais-Germain B: *Anatomie pour le Mouvement*. Meolans Revel: Editions Désiris; 1991

[33] Calais-Germain B: *Le Périnée Feminin*. Arques: Prodim; 1997

[34] Cambier J, Dehen H, Poirier J, Ribadeau-Dumas JL. *Propédeutique Neurologique*. Paris: Masson; 1976

[35] Cathie AG. *The Writings and Lectures of A.G. Cathie*. Indianapolis: AAO; 1974

[36] Ceccaldi A, Favre JF. *Les Pivots Ostéopathiques*. Paris: Masson; 1986

[37] Chaitow L. *Cranial Manipulation Theory and Practice*. Edinburgh: Churchill Livingstone; 2000

[38] Chaitow L. *Fibromyalgia Syndrome*. Edinburgh: Churchill Livingstone; 2000

[39] Chaitow L. *Maintaining Body Balance Flexibility and Stability*. Edinburgh: Churchill Livingstone; 2004

[40] Chaitow L. *Modern Neuromuscular Techniques*. Edinburgh: Churchill Livingstone; 1997

[41] Chaitow L. *Muscle Energy Techniques*. Edinburgh: Churchill Livingstone; 2001

[42] Chaitow L. *Palpation Skills*. Edinburgh: Churchill Livingstone; 2000

[43] Chaitow L. *Positional Release Techniques*. Edinburgh: Churchill Livingstone; 2002

[44] Chapman F. *An Endocrine Interpretation of Chapman's Reflexes*. Indianapolis: American Academy of Osteopathy; 1937

[45] Chauffour P, Guillot JM. *Le Lien Mécanique Ostéopathique*. Paris: Maloine; 1985

[46] Cole WV: *The Cole Book*. Indianapolis: AAO; n.d.

[47] Colot T, Verheyen M. *Manuel Pratique de Manipulations Ostéopathiques*. Paris: Maisonneuve; 1996

[48] De Wolf AN. *Het sacroiliacale Gewricht, Huidige inzichten Symposium 1.4.1989*. Utrecht: Smith Kline & French; 1990

[49] Di Giovanna E, Schiowitz S. *An Osteopathic Approach to Diagnosis and Treatment*. 2nd ed. Philadelphia: Lippincott-Raven; 1997

[50] Downing CH. *Osteopathic Principles in Disease*. Indianapolis: AAO; 1988

[51] Dummer T: *A Textbook of Osteopathy 1*. East Sussex: JoTom Publications; 1999

[52] Dummer T: *A Textbook of Osteopathy 2*. East Sussex: JoTom Publications; 1999

[53] Dummer T: *Specific Adjusting Technique*. East Sussex: JoTom Publications; 1995

[54] Feely RA. *Clinique Ostéopathique dans le Champ Crânien*. French translation by Louwette HO. Paris: Frison-Roche; 1988

[55] Finet G, Williame CH. *Biométrie de la Dynamique-Viscérale et Nouvelles Normalisations Ostéopathiques*. Paris: Les Editions Jollois; 1992

[56] Fryette HH. *Principes de la Technique Ostéopathique*. Translated by Abehsera A and Burty F. Paris: Frison-Roche; 1983

[57] Frymann VM. *The Collected Papers of Viola Frymann*. Indianapolis: AAO; 1998

[58] Füeßl F, Middeke M. *Duale Reihe Anamnese und klinische Untersuchung*. 2nd ed. Stuttgart: Thieme; 2002

[59] Gesret JR. *Asthme*. Paris: Editions de Verlaque; 1996

[60] Giammatteo T, Weiselfish-Giammatteo S. *Integrative Manual Therapy for the Autonomic Nervous System and Related Disorders*. Berkeley: North Atlantic Books; 1997

[61] Gleditsch JM: *Reflexzonen und Somatotopien*. Schorndorf: WBV; 1983

[62] Gray H. *Gray's Anatomie*. London: Pamajon; 1995

[63] Greenman P. *Lehrbuch der osteopathischen Medizin*. 3rd ed. Stuttgart: Haug; 2005

[64] Grieve GP. *Common Vertebral Joint Problems*. Edinburgh: Churchill Livingstone; 1988

[65] Grieve GP. *Mobilisation of the Spine*. Edinburgh: Churchill Livingstone; 1991

[66] Habermann-Horstmeier L. *Anatomie, Physiologie und Pathologie*. Stuttgart: Schattauer; 1992

[67] Handoll N: *Die Anatomie der Potency*. Pähl: Jolandos; 2004

[68] Hebgen E. *Vizeralosteopathie*. 2nd ed. Stuttgart: Hippokrates; 2005

[69] Helsmoortel J. *Lehrbuch der viszeralen Osteopathie*. Stuttgart: Thieme; 2002

[70] Hepp R, Debrunner H. *Orthopädisches Diagnostikum*. 7th ed. Stuttgart: Thieme; 2004

[71] Hoppenfeld S. *Examen Clinique des Membres et du Rachis*. Paris: Masson; 1984

[72] Jealous JS: *The Biodynamics of Osteopathy*. [CD ROMs]. Farmington: Biodynamics/Biobasics Program; 2002–2003

[73] Johnston WL. *Scientific Contributions of William L. Johnson*. Indianapolis: AAO; 1998

[74] Kapandji IA. *Physiologie Articulaire, Vols I–III*. Paris, Maloine; 1977

[74a] Kappler KA. *Postural balance and motion patterns*. J Am Osteopath Assoc. 1982; 81:598

[75] Kimberly PE. *Outline of Osteopathic Manipulative Procedures*. 3rd ed. Kirksville: Kirksville College of Osteopathic Medicine; 1980

[76] Kissling R. *Das Sacroiliacalgelenk*. Stuttgart: Enke; 1997

[76a] Klein KK, Redler I, Lowman CL. *Asymmetries of growth in the pelvis and legs of children: a clinical and statistical study 164–1967*. J Am Osteopath Assoc. 1968; 68:153

[77] Klein P, Sommerfeld P. *Biomechanik der menschlichen Gelenke*. Munich: Urban & Fischer; 2004

[78] Klinke R, Silbernagl S. *Lehrbuch der Physiologie*. Stuttgart: Thieme; 2003

[79] Korr IM. *The Collected Papers of Irvin M. Korr, Vols I and II*. Indianapolis: AAO; 1979, 1997

[80] Kramer J. *Bandscheibenbedingte Erkrankungen*. Stuttgart: Thieme; 1994

[81] Kuchera WA, Kuchera ML. *Osteopathic Considerations in Systemic Dysfunction*. Rev. 2nd ed. Columbus: Greyden Press; 1994

[82] Kuchera WA, Kuchera ML. *Osteopathic Principles in Practice*. Rev. 2nd ed. Columbus: Greyden Press; 1993

[83] Landouzy JM. *Les ATM Evaluation. Traitement Odontologiques et Ostéopathiques*. Paris: Editions de Verlaque; 1993

[84] Lee D. *The Pelvic Girdle*. Edinburgh: Churchill Livingstone; 1999

[85] Leonhardt M, Tillmann B, Tördury G, Zilles K. *Anatomie des Menschen. Lehrbuch und Atlas*. Stuttgart: Thieme; 2002

[86] Lewit K. *Lewit Manuelle Medizin*. 7th ed. Heidelberg: Barth; 1997

[86a] Lewit K. *Manipulative Therapy in Rehabilitation of the Locomotor System*. 3rd ed. Oxford: Butterworth–Heinemann; 1999

[87] Liebenson C. *Rehabilitation of the Spine*. Philadelphia: William and Wilkins; 1996

[88] Liem T, Dobler TK. *Leitfaden Osteopathie*. Munich: Urban & Fischer; 2002

[89] Liem T. *Kraniosakrale Osteopathie*. 3rd ed. Stuttgart: Hippokrates; 2001

[90] Liem T. *Praxis der Kraniosakralen Osteopathie*. 2nd ed. Stuttgart: Hippokrates; 2003

[91] Lignon A. *Le Puzzle Crânien*. Paris: Editions de Verlaque; 1989

[92] Lignon A. *Schématisation Neurovégétative en Ostéopathie*. Paris: Editions de Verlaque; 1987

[93] Lipincott RC, Lipincott HA. *A Manual of Cranial Technique*. Fort Worth: The Cranial Academy Inc.; 1995

[94] Littlejohn JM et al.: *Classical Osteopathy. Reprinted Lectures from the Archives of the Osteopathic Institute of Applied Technique*. Maidstone: The John Wernham College of Classical Osteopathy; n.d.

[95] Littlejohn JM: *Lesionology*. Maidstone: Maidstone College of Osteopathy; n.d.

[96] Littlejohn JM: *The Fundamentals of Osteopathic Technique*. London: BSO; n.d.

[97] Littlejohn JM: *The Littlejohn Lectures, Vol I*. Maidstone: Maidstone College of Osteopathy; n.d.

[98] Littlejohn JM. *The Pathology of the Osteopathic Lesion*. Maidstone College of Osteopathy. Indianapolis: AAO Yearbook; 1977

[99] McKenzie RA: *Die lumbale Wirbelsäule*. Waikanae: NZ Spinal Publications; 1986

[100] McKone WL. *Osteopathic Athletic Healthcare*. London: Chapman & Hall; 1997

[101] Magoun H. *Osteopathy in the Cranial Field*. Original ed. Fort Worth: SCTF, 2nd reprinting 1997

[102] Magoun H. *Osteopathy in the Cranial Field*. Fort Worth: SCTF; 1976

[103] Meallet S, Peyrière J. *L'Ostéopathie Tissulaire*. Paris: Editions de Verlaque; 1987

[104] Meert G. *Das Becken aus osteopathischer Sicht*. Munich: Urban & Fischer; 2003

[105] Milne M. *The Heart of Listening 1*. Berkeley: North Atlantic Books; 1995

[106] Milne M. *The Heart of Listening 2*. Berkeley: North Atlantic Books; 1995

[107] Mitchell FL Jr, Mitchel PKG: *The Muscle Energy Manual, Vols 1–2*. East Lansing; MET Press 2004

[108] Myers TW. *Anatomy Trains*. Munich: Urban & Fischer; 2004

[109] Netter F. *Farbatlanten der Medizin. Vol. 5 Nervensystem I, Neuroanatomie und Physiologie*. Stuttgart: Thieme; 1987

[110] Niethard F, Pfeil J. *Duale Reihe Orthopädie*. 3rd ed. Stuttgart: Thieme; 2003

[111] O'Connell JA. *Bioelectric Fascial Activation and Release*. Indianapolis: AAO; 1998

[112] Patterson MM, Howell JN. *The Central Connection: Somatovisceral/Viscerosomatic Interaction*. Indianapolis: AAO; 1992

[113] Peterson B. *Postural Balance and Imbalance*. Indianapolis: AAO; 1983

[114] von Piekartz H. *Kraniofasziale Dysfunktionen und Schmerzen*. Stuttgart: Thieme; 2000

[115] Pschyrembel: *Klinisches Wörterbuch*. Berlin: Walter de Gruyter; 2002

[116] Rauber/Kopsch (editors Tillmann B, Töndury G, Zilles K): *Anatomie des Menschen Vols I–IV*. 3rd ed. Stuttgart: Thieme; 2003

[117] Reibaud P. *Potentiel Ostéopathique Crânien, Mobilité Crânienne, Techniques Crâniennes*. Paris: Editions de Verlaque; 1990

[118] Ricard F, Thiebault P. *Les Techniques Ostéopathiques Chiropractiques Américaines*. Paris: Frison Roche; 1991

[119] Ricard F. *Traitement Ostéopathique des Douleurs d'Origine Lombo-Pelvienne, Vol 1*. Paris: Atman; 1988

[120] Ricard F. *Traitement Ostéopathique des Douleurs d'Origine Lombo-Pelvienne, Vol 2*. Paris: Atman; 1988

[121] Richard JP. *La Colonne Vertébrale en Ostéopathie, Vol 1*. Paris: Editions de Verlaque; 1987

[122] Richard R. *Lésions Ostéopathiques du Membre Inférieur*. Paris: Maloine; 1980

[123] Richard R. *Lésions Ostéopathiques du Sacrum*. Paris: Maloine; 1978

[124] Richard R. *Lésions Ostéopathiques Iliaques*. Paris: Maloine; 1979

[125] Richard R. *Lésions Ostéopathiques Vertébrales, Vol 1*. Paris: Maloine; 1982

[126] Richard R. *Lésions Ostéopathiques Vertébrales, Vol 2*. Paris: Maloine; 1982

[127] Rohen J. *Funktionelle Anatomie des Menschen*. Stuttgart: Schattauer; 1998

[128] Rohen J. *Funktionelle Anatomie des Nervensystems*. Stuttgart: Schattauer; 1994

[129] Rohen J. *Topographische Anatomie*. Stuttgart: Schattauer; 1992

[130] Rolf I. *Re-establishing the Natural Alignement and Structural Integration of the Human Body for Vitality and Well-being*. Rochester/VT: Healing Arts Press; 1989

[131] Sammut E, Searle-Barnes P. *Osteopathische Diagnose*. Munich: Pflaum; 2000

[132] Schulz L, Feitis R. *The Endless Web*. Berkeley: North Atlantic Books; 1996

[133] Sergueef N. *Die Kraniosakrale Osteopathie bei Kindern*. Kötzting: Verl. f. Osteopathie; 1995

[134] Silbernagl S, Despopoulos A. *Taschenatlas der Physiologie*. 6th ed. Stuttgart: Thieme; 2003

[135] Sills F. *Craniosacral Biodynamics, Vols I and II*. Berkeley: North Atlantics Books; 2004

[136] Solano R. *Le Nourisson, L'Enfant et L'Ostéopathie Crânium*. Paris: Maloine; 1986

[137] Speece C, Crow W. *Osteopathische Körpertechniken nach W.G. Sutherland: Ligamentous Articular Strain (LAS)*. Stuttgart: Hippokrates; 2003

[138] Spencer H: *Die ersten Prinzipien der Philosophie*. Pähl: Jolandos; 2004

[139] Steinrücken H. *Die Differentialdiagnose des Lumbalsyndroms mit klinischen Untersuchungstechniken*. Berlin: Springer; 1998

[140] Still AT: *Das große Still-Kompendium*. Pähl: Jolandos; 2002

[141] Struyf-Denis G. *Les Chaînes Musculaires et Articulaires*. Paris: ICTGDS; 1979

[142] Sutherland WG. *Contributions of Thought*. Fort Worth: Rudra Press; 1998

[143] Sutherland WG. *Teachings in the Science of Osteopathy*. Fort Worth: Sutherland Cranial Teaching Foundation; 1990

[144] Sutherland WG. *The Cranial Bowl*. 1st ed. Reprint. Fort Worth: Free Press Co.; 1994

[145] Travell J, Simons DG. *Myofascial Pain and Dysfunction. The Trigger Point Manual, Vols I–II*. 2nd ed. Philadelphia: Lippincott Williams & Wilkins; 1999

[146] Tucker C. *The Mechanics of Sports Injuries*. Oxford: Blackwell; 1990

[147] Typaldos S. *Orthopathische Medizin*. Kötzting: Verlag f. Ganzh. Med.; 1999

[148] Upledger JE, Vredevoogd JD. *Lehrbuch der Craniosacralen Therapie I*. 5th ed. Stuttgart: Haug; 2003

[149] Upledger JE. *Die Entwicklung des menschlichen Gehirns und ZNS—A Brain is Born*. Stuttgart: Haug; 2004

[150] Upledger JE. *Lehrbuch der Craniosacralen Therapie II: Beyond the Dura*. Stuttgart: Haug; 2002

[151] Vannier L. *La Typologie et ses Applications Thérapeutiques*. Boiron; 1989

[152] Villeneuve P, Weber B. *Pied, Equilibre & Mouvement*. Paris: Masson; 2000

[153] Villeneuve P. *Pied Equilibre & Rachis*. Paris: Frison-Roche; 1998

[154] Villeneuve P. *Pied, Equilibre & Posture*. Paris: Frison-Roche; 1996

[155] Vleeming A, Mooney V, Dorman T, Snijders C, Stoeckart R. *Movement, Stability and Low Back Pain*. Edinburgh: Churchill Livingstone; 1999

[156] Ward RC. *Foundations of Osteopathic Medicine*. Philadelphia: Williams & Wilkins; 1997

[157] Wernham J: *Osteopathy, Notes on the Technique and Practice*. Maidstone: Maidstone Osteopathic Clinic; 1975

[158] Willard FH, Patterson MM. *Nociception and the Neuroendocrine–Immune Connection*. Indianapolis: AAO; 1994

[159] Wodall P. *Principes et Pratique Ostéopathiques en Gynécologie*. Paris: Maloine; 1983

[160] Wright S. *Physiologie. Appliqué à la Médecine*. Paris: Flammarion; 1980

Trigger Points and Their Treatment (Hebgen)

[1] Baldry P. *Akupunktur, Triggerpunkte und muskuloskelettale Schmerzen.* 1st ed. Uelzen: Medizinisch Literarische Verlagsgesellschaft; 1993

[2] Dvořák J. *Manuelle Medizin—Diagnostik.* 4th ed. Stuttgart: Thieme; 2001

[3] Fleischhauer K (editor). *Benninghoff Anatomie: Makroskopische und mikroskopische Anatomie des Menschen—Vol 2.* 13th/14th eds. Munich: Urban & Schwarzenberg; 1985

[4] Klinke R, Silbernagl S (editors). *Lehrbuch der Physiologie.* 1st ed. Stuttgart: Thieme; 1994

[5] Kostopoulos D, Rizopoulos K. *The Manual of Trigger Point and Myofascial Therapy.* 1st ed. Thorofare: Slack Incorporated; 2001

[6] Kuchera ML. *Integrating Trigger Points into Osteopathic Approaches.* Berlin: IFAO-Fortbildung; 2004

[7] Kuchera ML, Kuchera WA. *Osteopathic Considerations in Systemic Dysfunction.* 2nd ed. Columbus: Greyden Press; 1994

[8] Lang F. *Pathophysiologie—Pathobiochemie.* 3rd ed. Stuttgart: Enke; 1987

[9] Netter FH. *Atlas der Anatomie des Menschen.* 2nd ed. Basel: Ciba-Geigy AG; 1994

[10] Pöntinen P, Gleditsch J, Pothmann R. *Triggerpunkte und Triggermechanismen.* 2nd ed. Stuttgart: Hippokrates; 2001

[11] Putz R, Pabst R (editors). *Sobotta: Atlas der Anatomie des Menschen—Vol 2.* 20th ed. Munich: Urban & Schwarzenberg; 1993

[12] Schmidt RF, Thews G (editors). *Physiologie des Menschen.* 29th ed. Berlin: Springer; 2004

[13] Schünke M, Schulte E, Schumacher U. *Prometheus—Lernatlas der Anatomie. Allgemeine Anatomie und Bewegungssystem.* 1st ed. Stuttgart: Thieme; 2004

[14] Schünke M. *Topographie und Funktion des Bewegungssystems.* 1st ed. Stuttgart: Thieme; 2000

[15] Schwegler J. *Der Mensch—Anatomie und Physiologie.* 3rd ed. Stuttgart: Thieme; 2002

[16] Silbernagl S, Despopoulos A. *Taschenatlas der Physiologie.* 3rd ed. Stuttgart: Thieme; 1988

[17] Simons D. *Myofascial Pain Syndrome Due to Trigger Points.* 1st ed. Cleveland: Gebauer Company; 1987

[18] Staubesand J (editor). *Benninghoff Anatomie: Makroskopische und mikroskopische Anatomie des Menschen—Vol 1.* 13th ed. Munich: Urban & Schwarzenberg; 1985

[19] Staubesand J (editor). *Sobotta: Atlas der Anatomie des Menschen—Vol 1.* 19th ed. Munich: Urban & Schwarzenberg; 1988

[20] Travell J, Simons D. *Myofascial Pain and Dysfunction – The Trigger Point Manual, Vol. 1.* 1st ed. Baltimore: Williams & Wilkins; 1983

[21] Travell J, Simons D. *Myofascial Pain and Dysfunction— The Trigger Point Manual, Vol. 2.* 1st ed. Baltimore: Williams & Wilkins; 1992

[22] Whitaker RH, Borley NR. *Anatomiekompaß: Taschenatlas der anatomischen Leitungsbahnen.* 1st ed. Stuttgart: Thieme; 1997

[23] Zenker W (editor). *Benninghoff Anatomie: Makroskopische und mikroskopische Anatomie des Menschen— Vol 3.* 13/14th eds. Munich: Urban & Schwarzenberg; 1985

Index

torsion 86
gait cycle 39–41
  biomechanics *40*
  stance stage 39–44, *40*, *42*, *43*
  swing stage 39–42, *40*
  weight shifts *41*, *42*, *43*
gastrocnemius 206, *207*
gluteus maximus *186*, 186–187, *187*
  dorsal chain 86
gluteus medius *187*, 187–188, *188*
gluteus minimus 188–189, *189*
gracilis muscle 196, *196*

H

hand(s) *165*, *167*, *169*
  flexion chain 82
head and neck pain 125–140
hip
  extension chain 84–85
  flexion chain 81
  limited extension 107
hip flexors *see* iliopsoas
hip pain 191–193, *192*
hip rotation test *102*
hip rotators *92*, 92–93
homeostasis 8
horizontal muscle chains 13–15
hormones, pain perception 32
hyoid bone *127*
  characteristics 92
hypertonicity 70, 77
  muscle energy technique 108
hypotonicity 70

I

iliac dysfunction, leg length 97
iliac fascia 91
iliacus muscle 183
iliocostal muscle 177
iliolumbosacral junction
  force neutralization 96
  posture 94, 96
iliopsoas 183–185
  characteristics *91*, 91–92
ilium
  extension chain 84–85
  flexion chain 81
infraspinatus muscle 144, *145*
inhalation 89–90
  peripheral bone movement *90*
  thoracic 56–57
  trunk movement *90*
intercostal muscles, trunk rotation 92
internal rotation 79
interosseus muscles (foot) 215, 217
interosseus muscles (hand) 168–170
intracranial membranes *46*, *47*
intraossal dysfunction 53–56
  cranial bone lesions 53
  occiput lesions 54–56
  skull base lesions 54
ischemic compression 122

ischiocrural muscles
  knee stretching 66
  patient examination *104*
isolytic muscle energy technique 108
isometric contraction 108
isotonic concentric contraction 108
isotonic eccentric contraction 108

J

joint normalization, muscle energy technique 107, 108

K

Kabat, Herman, proprioceptive neuromuscular
  facilitation 10–11
knee
  extension chain 85
  flexion chain 81
knee pain 200–202, *201*
knee stretching
  ischiocrural muscles *see* ischiocrural muscles
  quadriceps 66
Korr, Irvin M., 34–36
  locomotor system 4
  nervous system 36
kypholordosis 7, 11
  gait 39
  treatment 96

L

latent trigger points 113
lateral line 16, *17*
lateral pterygoid muscle 131, *131*
lateral strain 3, 53
latissimus dorsi 146–147, *147*
  dorsal chain 86
  patient examination *104*
left pectoralis major, ventral chain 86
leg length differences 97–100
  correction 99
  diagnosis 98–99
  musculoskeletal system effects 97–98
  symptoms 97–98
Le Lien Mécanique en Osteopathie (The Mechanical
  Link in Osteopathy) 25–26
lemniscates, stability 77–78
levator ani muscle 185–186
levator scapulae 140, *141*, *142*
Littlejohn, John Martin
  gait 43
  pivots *see* pivots
  biomechanics of the spine *see* spinal column
locomotor system 4
  biomechanics 7
  composition 5
  respiratory movement 89–91
longissimus muscle 178
Lovett's Laws 37
lower crossed syndrome *69*, 70
lower leg pain 202–219
lower thoracic aperture